Intermittent Fasting

Shortcut to Build Muscle, Lose Fat and Easy Weight Loss

Brian Adams

© Copyright 2015 - All rights reserved.

Brian Adams

Table of Contents

Introduction

Throughout the years, we've always been told that to lose weight we should start the day with a healthy breakfast. Why? Because our metabolism needs a much needed boost to start the day. The old saying springs to mind – "Breakfast like a king, lunch a prince and dinner like a pauper." But how much truth is there in this?

Well, the next thing you hear is, if you really want to lose weight then eat several small meals throughout the day instead of three. This keeps your metabolism working at optimum levels all day. Again, how much truth is there in this?

What I am going to show you will turn this on its head. I am going to show you how intermittent fasting is actually the way to lose weight, not eating so many times a day and at certain times. If you want to lose weight safely and be healthy then follow the advice in this eBook – you won't regret it; I promise.

This book may prove to be a turnaround for those of you who have found themselves going on all the diets out there trying to stabilize their weight. I know all about the effect of yoyo dieting. I come from a family of overweight people. We always blamed it on our genes. It was only when I started intermittent fasting that I realized it was nothing of the kind and you can only go on blaming something like this for so long. You have to learn which fasting type works for you, but when you do, you actually feel energized and on a high. I did and I am not able to keep to a regular weight and build up muscle. My body is eating into my fat all of the time I am writing this. Why? Because this is the window within my day when I choose not to eat.

There are all kinds of advice out there on fasting and dieting but what makes this book different is that someone who practices what they preach and knows all of the pitfalls and the weaknesses of the people who try this change in their routine writes it. I also know what it's like to feel so overweight that I had trouble walking up a hill. That told me that something was wrong and it was time I fixed it. The blame was clearly on me, and like me, you cannot pass responsibility on to someone or something else for the rest of your life.

Fasting will help you to find that balance in your life. It is easier than dieting and more effective and the routine, once set, is very easy to incorporate into your life. This book also contains a chart to my secret weapon against weight gain, which will help you to decide upon the best intermittent fasting system to incorporate into your day-to-day living. Once you do, your body gets a chance to heal itself correctly and you can also get rid of sluggish digestion problems and constipation. I used to blame that on slow metabolism but it wasn't. It was because of my eating habits. Change with me and try it out because long-term, your body will thank you for it, and you may even live a longer! That's the bonus to this style of eating and caring for your body.

Brian Adams

What is Intermittent Fasting?

I must make this clear – intermittent fasting is NOT a diet. Instead, it is a conscious decision that you make to skip out certain meals. It also does not mean starving yourself. What it entails is a kind of feast and fast – all your daily calories are eaten during a certain part of the day and then you do not eat anything else for the rest of the day.

There are two main ways that you can do this:

- Pick a specific window of time and stick to it regularly. For example, choose to eat from noon to 8 pm only, thus skipping breakfast and not eating after 8 pm. Some choose a 4 or 6-hour window, so it's whatever suits you.

Here is a chart that I live by. I chose the first option here because it wasn't hard for me at all. Instead of having breakfast in the morning, I have breakfast at noon. It doesn't matter what time of day you have it so why not? In fact, I actually enjoy my food more and appreciate that breakfast for the first time in my life. There was always a begrudging feeling attached to being forced to eat before I went to work. Now I don't have to do that anymore and, as it was my nature not to eat breakfast naturally it followed that this was the easiest method for me, and probably will be for most people. The hardest bit is knowing that you can't snack in the evening, but you soon get used to that time frame and it's a lot easier than the alternatives.

Day and Hour	Monday	Tuesday	Weds.	Thurs.	Friday	Sat.	Sunday
8pm/midday							
Midday							
3pm							
6pm							
7 pm							
8pm							
Fasting period	Light eating		Small Meal		Main Meal		

This fasting chart is what I have stuck to my fridge door. I actually don't need it there anymore because I am so accustomed to this way of life that it isn't a hardship for me. I don't feel like I am depriving myself of anything because I never liked breakfast anyway and most of the time that I am fasting, I am asleep.

The worst thing about this when you start is the fact that you have to do without your morning coffee if you like milk in coffee. I forced myself to drink black coffee and to drink more water and it's really helped because I never drank much water in the past, which probably contributed, to my sluggish digestion. If you suffer from constipation, it's probably because of this. I know in my case it was and that problem is a problem of the past now.

What few people appreciate is that during the hours of sleep, your body is still burning calories. If it has less calories to burn then it will eat into the fat stores and you will lose weight much more easily. I used to be a person who didn't sleep well and I have found that I actually look forward to sleep on the intermittent fasting regime because sleep is the way to get through one fasting period to the next without actually craving food. If you think that you may have difficulty getting through the day without eating, this is probably the best choice for you because you can still have two meals in a day and lose weight. Plus, you don't have to be totally anti-social and go into long explanations to friends about being on a fast.

- Cut out 2 meals every day. For example, eat as normal and finish your last meal at 8 pm then don't eat the following day until 8 pm. That gives you a full 24-hour without eating.

Day and Hour	Monday	Tuesday	Weds.	Thurs.	Friday	Saturday	Sunday
8pm							
Night							
Breakfast							
Lunch							

Now, I dare say at this point you are thinking to yourself that skipping a meal or two sounds easy and that you will lose weight. Why? Because you are eating less calories. Well, that is true but only partly. By cutting one meal from your day, you can eat more at the other meals but still consume fewer calories per day. And less calories is equal to losing weight, right?

Not necessarily. Not all calories are the same, they are not treated equally, and, what is more important is the time at which you eat. Bear in mind that the later you eat, the more chance there is of food not digesting properly, unless you are intending to go to the gym late at night or go for a jog at 1 am.

The earlier you eat, the more active you are and the more chance you have of burning off the calories you do eat. In the next chapter, I am going to explain how this all works. The above chart is the 24 hour fast but it's hard to keep to unless you are going through a period of training. Personally, it isn't a great long-term solution because it's anti-social and means you have to explain to people why you cannot eat on certain days and it's difficult because there are too many variances.

Those who do use this system tend to lose a steady amount of weight, but it's likely that the deprivation will be felt. 24 hours is quite a long time to go without food and you need real discipline to use this system, whereas the one that I suggest is a much easier regime to follow. The 24-hour fasting can be done intermittently through the week, thus having two days when you don't eat instead of every other day. You need to change your attitude toward eating if you choose to use this system because you must consider it a way of life rather than just a temporary way to lose a little weight. The problem is you get into the area of the yoyo diet if you view it in any other way. The moment you decide fasting isn't for you, your body goes back to being sluggish and the old habits creep in again.

You can see from this that my way makes much better sense. I don't eat until lunchtime and I don't eat after 8 in the evening. That makes it clear cut and much easier because I can still have lunch with friends and coffee with them in the afternoons. I just avoid social gatherings in the mornings or stick to black coffee and am not tempted by cakes that I am offered because my regime is very strict and is for the rest of my life. In fact, even in hospital recently for something which was not digestion related, I was able to keep to my fast with absolutely no interruption or complaints from the nursing staff.

Since I expended less energy in hospital, it also meant that I wasn't allowing myself to eat huge meals. The hospital food made sure of that, and after meals, I tended to exercise a little because it helps the healing process anyway and it's not good to lie in bed prolonging the hospital stay.

Thus, of the suggested fasting regimes, I still swear that mine is the best choice. It's certainly the easiest choice to make and fits in with modern lifestyle without me having to explain to everyone that I am on any kind of diet at all. I do find that I drink a lot more water than I used to but that's a good thing because it helps the hydration of the body and my skin is so fresh, whereas before it was a little patchy and difficult to keep looking fresh.

So to sum it up for you, here is a condensation of the above.

Intermittent fasting is not a diet. Don't confuse it to help you lose weight radically like a crash diet would. It is meant to help you lose weight gradually and you will have the body of your dreams ultimately. The intermittent fasting technique is meant to be a slightly slow process and you are not rushed to see any results. So understand the distinction between the two processes before you decide to take up intermittent fasting.

This fasting technique is meant to help you remain fit and healthy for long. So the basic idea is for you to convert this fast into a lifestyle choice and not merely take it up as a fancy diet that will make you lose weight before a beauty contest. It is meant to be a sustainable activity that will allow you to remain fit and healthy for a long time. The fasting is meant to help your body adjust to the new habits so that you don't feel like going back to your old habits.

The intermittent fasting technique is designed to help your body burn the excess calories and not store any new fat in your body. As you know, we end up eating a lot of calorific foods in a day and that is what the intermittent fast tackles. It ensures that you don't consume calorific foods and help your body burn away the fat that already exists. So it is like a double action technique where you don't add in any more calorific foods and assist in burning away any existing fat in your body.

The basic design of the diet is to give your body the chance to burn the calories that you ate during the meal. If you keep subjecting it to one calorific meal after another, you will only confuse your body. It is important that you leave sufficient gap between two or meals for your body to burn away the fat easily. You will realize that you are much fitter and active after you start on the diet. So weight loss is not the only goal of the diet and also incorporates your fitness.

Ideally, you must cut 2 meals in a day. These will depend on how long your body takes to break down the calories. Most people prefer to cut out their breakfast and maybe a snack in between. So that leaves you with your lunch and dinner. This will ensure that there is enough time for your body to burn the calories and also help you remain active and alert all through the day.

Apart from the food, water is also an important part of the fast. You have to drink at least 8 glasses of water a day if you wish to flush out all the unnecessary toxins from your body. You will also not feel constipated and remain full of energy. Many people forget to consume water regularly and say that they are extremely busy and forget about it. So the best thing to do is carry a bottle wherever you go and force yourself to drink a little every now and then.

Skipping meals is one of the main aspects of the diet and you must understand that it is meant to be a safe option. We have all grown up knowing that skipping meals, especially breakfast, is a bad health choice to make, but it is fine to do so provided you know what to skip and when to do so. Don't make a timetable of your own and come up with one that is carefully crafted. You will know your body best and it will be a good idea to create the meal plan by yourself.

Remember that the diet will work differently for everyone. So don't compare your progress with that of others. It will work for you too but you must remain patient. Expecting to see quick results is not possible. You have to take it slow and allow your body to adjust to the diet. Pushing yourself is not the way forward. Remain persistent and you will see positive results.

If any of these problems bug you, then my way is probably the right way for you to go:

Constipation, self-discipline and skin problems.

Brian Adams

History of Fasting

Fasting has existed since time immemorial. There was a time when people relied only on fasting to help them regain strength from an illness. Researchers believe that it is not possible to point out exactly when fasting might have come about. It might have occurred during the early days of man's existence or come about later.

But since man has existed for millions of years, it is safe to assume early man himself started the concept of fasting and it has manifested itself in many forms since. So the basic motive of man might not have been to lose weight and build muscles and instead, help the body recuperate from an illness and induce strength. Life was tough for man before where he had to bear extreme weather conditions and there were no super markets to pick up food. He had to hunt and gather and many times, there would be no food available. So in one sense, he would end up fasting, as he would have no access to any food.

Apart from this reason, most organisms are designed by god to go into a phase of dieting to help regain strength and vigor. So not just man but also animals that existed a long time back indulged in fasting as a means to increase their strength and vigor.

Once man started to lead civilized lives, many other factors started affecting his food habits. Religion was one such factor that proved to be a strong influence. People started fasting by citing religious reasons and that is still a rampant practice amongst several religions.

Food was viewed as a gift to mankind and by sacrificing it he was sacrificing a valuable gift. It was also implemented as a means to break the bad habit of gluttony and prevent people from treating good food as a thorough necessity.

Yogis, who associated fasting with attaining good health, then adopted it. They believed that it was possible for people to not just detoxify their body but also give it a chance to process the different elements that are already present internally. So along with all the different poses that are meant to cleanse the organs, fasting and consuming water were seen as being the best solution to recuperate.

Modern day meaning of fasting, however, has changed drastically. People these days fast not because they are interested in remaining fit but wish to out do each other and turn skinny. Fasting is now better known as dieting and every other person you know will be on one diet or the other. This is completely ruining the very essence of fasting and making it look like a villain.

What's more, it is being used as a means to make money and commercial establishments are exploiting people by recommending one form of diet or the other. So the need of the hour is to differentiate fasting from dieting.

I'm sure you have already experienced several ill effects of these sporadic diets that people take up when they hear about someone else having benefitted from it. We humans will go to any extent to fit into society regardless of whether or not it is ideal for our body. So it is important to separate fact from fiction and reevaluate our opinions.

But it is easier said than done as people have pre formed notions about dieting. They will assume that the diet is meant to make them lose weight fast and maintain a skinny body with less mass. But that is not what fasting is meant to do. Fasting is a technique used to help the body remain healthy and get rid of unnecessary toxins.

Brian Adams

Fasting is a great tool that you can use to holistically improve your body's functions increasing metabolism. But you have to understand the right way of doing it to know whether or not you are doing the right thing. There is enough scientific evidence to prove it and it has been established how those taking up regular fasts are in a position to combat several common illnesses. That is why many holistic and alternate medicine gurus prescribe fasting as a means to increase your immunity and strengthen your body. You can also remain full of energy and not have to worry about not having some by the end of the day.

The intermittent fasting is a technique where the person restricts his or her calorie intake and focuses on a fasting and non-fasting form of diet. Although it is meant to help in lose weight, it also assists in building a strong body with strong bones.

In this book, we will look at the intermittent diet in detail and explore its various facets. We will also read on supplementary activities that you must take up to help the intermittent fast work better.

How Does Intermittent Fasting Work?

Your body reacts differently when you feast, compared to when you fast. When you eat, your body needs to take a few hours out to digest and process your food. It will burn off what it can and, under a "normal" diet, the rest is stored as fat – depending on what you eat. However, when you are in an intermittent fast, your body uses all this readily available fuel, rather than going to the fat stores in your body. You see, your body will take the easy way out and burn what's already in your bloodstream, especially if what you ate had sugar or a high carbohydrate content. The human body is used to burning carbohydrate as its main source of fuel and, if it's there and readily available, it will use it over and above fat stores.

Now, when you fast, your body cannot call on recently eaten food to burn so it can only turn to your fat stores for energy, rather than any glycogen in your muscles or glucose that is in your blood stream. And, as we all know, burning fat means losing weight and that's a win in anyone's book. I know that at first, I was disappointed with the slowness of the results, but little by little I began to notice muscle building up and toning of my body around the stomach area. This was an area where I had not, for example, felt my hipbones for years. They always had a layer of fat over them. Now, I can feel them and see the contours of this area much more clearly. Instead of having to hide away in clothing that was loose to hide the flab, I can now wear more tailored clothing and look good. That's got to make a huge difference to people who are overweight and who have been looking for solutions.

The same goes for if you go for a workout or a run when you are in a fasting period. Because your body doesn't have that supply of sugar, or glucose to call on, because you haven't replaced it by eating, then it has to adapt and pull the energy it needs from fat stores in your cells. Thus, any exercise that you do, no matter how sedentary, is going to help you to lose fat. Walking, skipping, cycling and even circling the house in a fast walk all helped me to lose fat.

Why does this work? When we eat, our body reacts by producing a chemical called insulin. The more sensitivity you have towards insulin, the more likely you are to make efficient use of the food that you consume and that leads to a loss of weight and the creation of muscle tissue. And, if you didn't already know, your body is at its most insulin-sensitive after a period of fasting.

Glycogen is a starch that is stored in your liver and your muscles. The body can use it as energy if it needs to but, more often than not, it will disappear overnight – or when you fast. And, if you train hard or go to a gym on a regular basis, it will be even further depleted and that ups your insulin sensitivity even more. What this means is that eating straight after a workout means your body will process the food far more efficiently – most of the food will be stored as glycogen in the muscles, burned immediately as energy to help your body recover and, what little is left stored as fat. Thus, at the end of the morning, I tend to do my workout. I call it a workout, but if you adopt the same attitude as me, it's fun rather than punishment. I have this system of workout that suits my lifestyle and simply lock myself away from the world and put on a dance video and do Zumba. It doesn't matter how good I am at it. What matters is that it becomes a regular part of my life just before the fasting is over. That's easy for me because the video lasts less than 20 minutes and I don't have to explain to people where I am disappearing off. You can use any kind of exercise you like, but this works well for me and doesn't seem like punishment to my body. You really need to find something that you enjoy if you decide to go for an intermittent fasting regime so that you don't feel deprived at all and you still feel like you are having fun out of life. I feel so much more energized and my dance routine is getting rather good.

Now compare this to a day of your normal diet. You know, where you eat those 3 or 6 meals a day and possibly even snack in between as well. Because your sensitivity to insulin is at normal levels, the carbohydrates and the glucose in the food you eat will see that your glycogen stores are already full to bursting; that you already have plenty of glucose in your blood and will head straight to the fat stores where it will settle quite nicely, prepared to hunker in for the long haul! That's why people who are obese tend to get diabetes. There is just too much sugar in their bodies and the body can't cope with that amount of sugar. Thus, exercise just before eating helps considerably because the body will eat up all of the goodness from your fat stores.

On top of all that, when you fast, your body produces a much higher level of growth hormone, and this is both after that period of fasting and while you are sleeping. Add to that increase the decrease in production of insulin, which leads to an increase in insulin sensitivity and your body, is primed and ready for muscle growth and losing fat when you go on an intermittent fast. For me, it's become a way of life. I am not deprived of anything at all. I just don't eat between 8 at night and midday and that's a pretty easy rule to stick to. It makes less work too so I have more time to do things that I enjoy doing.

In a nutshell, intermittent fasting teaches your body how to use the food you consume in a much more efficient manner and, done properly, it can promote weight loss and muscle growth. In my case, I have lost an awful lot of excess weight. I don't get puffed out any more and when my food is prepared, I really do enjoy it and sit down and celebrate eating it, rather than eating a quick sandwich on the go and not even knowing what was in the sandwich. Look at your lifestyle. You probably eat a lot of junk food. If you're going to eat under this regime, take your time eating and be aware of all the tastes and textures. When you eat slowly and appreciate what you eat you also stop yourself from getting indigestion and all the indigestion related illnesses. Even my hiatus hernia doesn't play up any more.

Now it is obvious that you will need evidence to believe that the intermittent fast actually works. Apart from my experiences of being on the diet, you will need evidence of a scientific nature to believe that fasting really does work.

Well, there have been many scientists who have studied the intermittent diet carefully to understand whether or not it actually does work for people. They have successfully established evidence that proves how the diet works by modifying the internal metabolism of people.

As you know, the human body performs a complex set of functions that is difficult to understand and interpret. There are just so many things that are going on that it is impossible to understand each of them and know how to better them.

Without understanding these things fully, people decide to take up diets to lose their weight. They don't understand that it is not as simple as starving yourself, gaining an ideal weight and sticking with the diet. That only happens in movies and cartoons.

It is important to take up regular fasts, which will allow your body to adjust to it as opposed to resist it. When you take up a new diet, you will notice a few changes at the very beginning and then go back to square one. In fact, if not done the right way, then you will end up in a worse situation than when you started out.

So you have to understand the science behind a diet before you decide to take it up. It is understandable that most diets that are prescribed have a scientific backing and they are available on the Internet.

However, through regular research, scientists have established that the intermittent fasting technique is best suited for the human body. The diet is designed in such a way that, the eating matches the circadian rhythm of the body. So, everything in your body will be in sync and the food you in take will be welcomed easily. This is not possible if you keep filling up your body with food as and when you feel like doing it. You have to give your body the chance to adjust to a new routine and it will only get easier if you follow a set rhythm to do so.

Scientists have also established that this diet aids in eliminating unnecessary toxins from the body. So you are helping your body by getting rid of those things that are eating away from the inside. This diet therefore leaves you with other benefits such as glowing skin and shinier mane. We will look at these in detail in a future chapter.

So all in all, not only is this diet being lauded by the thousands of people, worldwide, who have seen a tremendous change in their health but also by scientists who have conducted due research on this topic and have established scientific evidence to back their claims.

Brian Adams

Why Not 5 Or 6 Small Meals Every Day?

A lot of diet books will tell you that you should eat several small meals a day rather than just 3 main ones. Some of the main reasons why they say this are:

- It takes calories to burn off the food you eat so it kind of makes sense that the more you eat, the more calories you burn. And if you eat small meals all day long, your body is burning calories all day long, and your body is on prime time permanently, yes?

- No. It really doesn't matter whether you eat 2000 calories in a while day or within a space of 4 hours, it takes the same amount of calories to process that food so you are not gaining anything by eating all day except for weight.

The logic behind the small meals regular is flawed. People use this as an excuse to eat all the wrong things, justifying what they eat by saying that they are only eating a small amount of it at a time, but it all adds up and the body doesn't have the time to process the food before the next lot of food is added. Thus, no matter how much people may find this popular myth fits with their lifestyle, it's a case of accepting that if you eat more, you give your body more calories and sooner or later, it's going to catch up with you. How do I know? I come from a family of fatties. We all have our problems and we all try to deal with them in our own ways. My sisters have tried all the diets in the book and not one of them has had the results that I have because they simply can't get their heads around fasting.

The problem is that if you think of it as deprivation, you tend to binge between fasting and that's counter-productive. I remember my sister eating a huge meal after her first fast and finishing off the meal with two doughnuts! This kind of compensation isn't positive at all. Why two? She could have left the doughnut until her three o'clock break and had it with a coffee and appreciated it. Instead she chose to pig out when the fast finished each day and then wondered why the fast hadn't worked for her.

- If you eat smaller meals then you won't eat too much on your main meal, right? There could be some truth in that, one of those who have a bit of a problem with portion control or if you don't really know how much you should be eating. However, all this takes especially if you are is a bit of education and you taking control of your food, not the other way around.

- To be fair, most people who eat 6 times a day find it somewhat prohibitive and it does take quite a lot of effort to do it. And, because you are eating several smaller meals, you probably never really feel full and that makes it more likely that you will eat more calories with every meal.

The only circumstances I can see this working is where you have a small stomach and can't manage large amounts of food, but in this case, you won't need to fast because your body is already lean. I say this because my partner is lean and has a very small stomach. He cannot eat a full meal and invariably leaves a lot of what is on his plate because he doesn't have room for it. In a case like this, where weight gain is not the problem, it's probably a good idea to eat small amounts regularly to keep up the energy levels, but if you are looking to lose weight and build up muscle instead of fat, it's not the most sensible diet to be on, especially bearing in mind that you will probably over compensate with the wrong types of food.

So, although the theory of little and often seems to be grounded in logic, it really doesn't work unless you do struggle with the amount of food you eat in one go. Now, go back to the caveman days. If they had needed to eat every three hours, they would have even in trouble. Let's face it, the caveman didn't exactly have a pocket watch he could pull out and check the time on. He ate what he could when he could and that meant fasting periods when he couldn't find anything to eat. They functioned and they suffered with far less obesity and health problems that we do today.

Of course, there's also the caveman diet to consider, but believe me, my sisters and I tried it and it's darned hard work. You have to use products that are not easy to find and go without flour and that's a real hassle. This diet works for me because there is no work attached to it. You simply do not eat between the hours of 8 in the evening until 12 the next day. What's hard about that?

Just recently, there have been a number of studies that prove the theory of "small and often" is wrong. Your see, the premise is that eating more leads to better regulation of the appetite and better dietary compliance. Plus, there has always been the thought that increasing the frequency of meals leads to better gut peptide profiles, which would lead to more weight loss. The studies rejected this completely, instead saying that it is not how much you eat, it is the quality and the type of food you are eating that counts.

I love my food. I don't deprive myself of anything, but I also don't pig out. Fresh salads are my favorite because there's so much flexibility. Add different vegetables each day, add a boiled egg or lean meat. I even have salads that I can prepare in minutes with the use of pasta. You don't have to deprive yourself. You can actually make eating a real joy as I do and still lose weight easily. It's actually a family joke that we eat at each other's houses regularly and compare diets. My sisters are always amazed at the variety of foods that I eat and haven't even tried some of the fruit and vegetables that I eat. I cut out potato a long time ago, because I knew that the starch wasn't doing me any good, but I do break this habit occasionally to have new potatoes cooked in water with mint because they are so delicious, but I make sure that the portion is relatively small and that it is eaten with other great vegetables that give me all the vitamins and minerals that I need.

Brian Adams

Why Should I Choose Intermittent Fast?

Because it works? Because it's simple? Why not? Let's look at the most basic reasons for choosing intermittent fasting as a way of losing weight.

- Because it works – we know that calories are not all the same but restricting them still plays a huge role in weight loss. When you go through a fasting period, whether it is for 16 hours every day or for 24 hours every few days, you are making it much easier on yourself to restrict those calories over the course of an entire week. His gives your body that chance it needs to shed some of those pounds, simply because you are eating less calories than you were before.

- It's simple – instead of having to prepare several meals in a day, you can simply skip a couple and only have to worry about preparing what you need for your eating window. I love this part because although I am basically a foodie, I hate the preparation and the kitchen is my least favorite room in the house. This way, from 8 at night, the kitchen is out of bounds to me so if anyone creates dirty dishes, it's their problem to clean up and I have even trained the kids to clean up their breakfast dishes. Life is easier for me.

- It takes less – time and money! Instead of having to make several meals, and buy the ingredients for them, every day, you only need to make two meals. Instead of stopping every few hours to eat, you only have to stop twice. Instead of having to wash up several times, it's only twice. See where I'm going? Even the kids asked if they could try it. I made the decision that until they were old enough to make decisions for themselves, then keeping to a normal diet was probably more beneficial for growing kids. However, my eldest daughter has joined me and with her keep fit regime and the intermittent fasting, it's likely that she won't follow in our family footsteps and become a biggie.

- Better sensitivity to insulin, and better growth hormone production, both of which are needed for weight loss.

Do you need any more reasons? It works; it's as simple as that. In the next chapter, I want to go over 5 of the most popular protocols of intermittent fasting. Even though my protocol works best for me, it may not be the best one for you. Thus, it's important to know the options available to everyone so that each person can choose according to their own circumstances. If you live an average lifestyle like me, you will find my choice the easiest option because most of the fasting period is spent in sleeping and that means I don't have to worry about it. However, look at the other choices and choose one that suits your lifestyle instead of taking my word for it.

Brian Adams

FAQ's On Intermittent Fasting

Now it is obvious that you will have a few doubts about the intermittent diet, as it is a new subject for you. In this chapter, we will look at the most common questions that get asked on the topic and answer them to help you understand the topic better.

Is it safe?

Yes. The intermittent diet is a safe option for you to take up. Intermittent fasting is meant to help you lose weight and also gain lean muscles. The intermittent diet is devised to help the body eliminate toxins and prepare it to undertake exercises that will help sculpt the body. The diet has existed for a long time and has been tried and tested by many people and so, you will not be the first one to take it up. It is an effective diet meant to help you remain fit and healthy for long and so, is a great diet for you to take up.

Is it for anyone?

Yes. The diet is safe for anyone interested in losing weight and increasing healthy muscles. As you know, muscles replace fat and prevent fat formation in the body. So by taking up the diet, you are cutting out on the unnecessary calories and increasing the muscle in your body. There is a restriction on the age and it is best for people above the age of 18 to take up the diet. The upper age limit will depend on the person's physicality and fitness level. In any case, it is best to consult the physician before taking up the diet and ensuring that your body is fit enough to take it up.

Is it difficult to take up?

Not really. The intermittent fast is not a diet as such and is only a schedule for a diet. So it is not difficult to take it up and you must make only a few changes in your existing diet. But before that, you must choose a fasting period for yourself like 16 hours or 24 hours and then stick with it. Whatever you choose, ensure that you do your research on the topic and only then take it up. Don't go into a diet without conducting due research and make sure that you are fully aware of what you are getting into.

Will it really work?

Yes. The intermittent fast has both scientific backing and testimonials from thousands of people who have tried the fast and availed its various benefits. The diet is said to be one of the best that you can choose for your body and mind to feel rejuvenated. The rules of this fast are not too strict and flexible enough for you to make any modifications. These modifications will ensure that you feel completely at ease and remain within your limits. That's what makes this fast unique and you will see results from it in no time at all.

Will it be permanent?

Yes. The results that you see from the diet will be permanent and so will be the diet. You can continue with it for as long as you like and never stop with it. It should be converted into a lifestyle choice and not a mere habit that you take up and exploit until you get bored of it. You efforts should be potent enough for you to take the diet seriously and stick with it for a lifetime. Remember that it will be completely up to you and you alone can make it a permanent habit if you put your mind to it.

How long will results take to show?

That depends on you and your physique. Different people will see different results at different times. So there is no telling when you will see positive results and when someone else will see theirs. But if you put in efforts and are really determined about it then you can see results within a month or so. But that does not mean you try it for a month and give up on it. The initial results will also be less but the progress will be cumulative. So remain determined to continue with the habit for as long as you can.

Will I feel tired?

No. If you follow the diet correctly then you will not feel tired. If you are doing something wrong then you might feel tired and fatigued. You have to calculate the calories that you take in and burn every day and work with numbers. That will ensure you don't feel tired and do all the right things for your body. But if you do feel tired then assess your diet plan and ask your doctor whether you are doing something wrong and fix it at the earliest.

Can I choose any type?

Yes. The type of intermittent fast you choose depends on you. You can pick the one that suits you the best. Although you can instantly know which one will work for you and which one might not, it is best to take all of them up one after the other and stick with the one that works best for your body. The ultimate goal of the diet is to help you lose weight and maintain the ideal weight as also build strong and lean muscles that are not easily burnt away. So as long as these needs are met, you can choose the diet of your choice.

Can I combine them?

Yes. You can combine two or more of these diets but ensure that you get it right. You can consult an expert on the topic to help you out and know what will work for you and what will not. The basic idea is to derive maximum benefit from the diet and ensure that you pick the one that suits your body type the best. If you think a combination will work best for you then you may pursue it.

Can I stop whenever?

Yes. Stopping is up to you but it is best to stop systematically. Don't give up on it abruptly and all too sudden. Take your time and allow your body to get adjusted to the changes. However, it is best to continue with the fast for a long time and not give up in it easily.

These form the various FAQs that get asked on the topic and hope you had yours answered efficiently.

Brian Adams

The Top 5 Intermittent Fasting Protocols

You may think that intermittent fasting is a simple method of just not eating but there is a right and a wrong way to do it. And there are also a number of protocols to choose from and getting the right one for you is vital if you really want to reap the benefits. So, without further ado, let's talk about the top 5 protocols:

16-hour Fast

This method is best for those who are dedicated to the gym and who want to build up muscle and lose fat.

How does it work? 14 hour fast for women and 16 hours for men every day. The remaining 6-8 hours are your "feast" time. During your fasting period, you must consume no calories whatsoever, although you may drink black coffee, diet soda, use calorie-free sweeteners and eat sugar-free gum. If you want a splash of milk in your drink, that isn't going to hurt you, either but if you are already overweight, avoid it.

Most people who choose this method find it easier to do this over the night and the morning. They eat their first meal around 6 hours after waking – incidentally, this is why your first meal is called breakfast – it is the meal that breaks your fast.

This is an easy protocol to fit into any schedule but you must maintain a consistent feast window of time. This is so that your hormones settle down and to make it easier to stick at it. What you eat also depends on your level of activity. On days that you exercises you should eat more carbohydrates than fat but on the days where you don't exercise, fat is more important. You should eat a high level of protein every single day though how much depends on a number of factors, such as age, weight, your goals, how much body fat you have and how active you are.

This is my choice and is shown in the first chart in a previous chapter. It's easy. It's fun. However, do get a balanced diet during the hours that you eat. I eat loads of fish and salads. I eat cheese and I eat Omega 3 rich foods because they always make me feel healthier. I tend not to be a very active person, but I make the effort now by walking, cycling (short distances), dancing and playing tennis. Thus I keep myself relatively active because that's important too.

Pros: - for the most part, you can eat whenever you want during your feast window although it may help if you break your food into three meals. In my case, I break it into breakfast, an afternoon tea and an evening meal. It's the easiest of all the plans because there are no real questions. You don't have to keep consulting a chart or calorie count. You just eat during your eating times.

Cons: - While when you eat is flexible, what you eat isn't. You cannot pig out on whatever you fancy because that would defeat the entire object. You must stick to a nutritionally balanced plan scheduled around your workouts. This was the hardest part of the program for me. I didn't exercise much but I did find that investing in a jump rope was a good idea as I actually enjoy skipping. If you can find some form of exercise that you like, for example swimming, then add this to your daily routine and you really will shape up fast.

24-hour Fast

This is the perfect plan for people who already eat healthily but want that extra push.

How does it work? This plan requires you to fast for a straight 24 hours one to two times every week. During that 24-hour period, you must eat nothing but you may consume drinks that are calorie free. After the 24 hours is up, you can go back to eating your normal diet. You can start the 24 hours whenever it suits you – some people prefer to end it at a main mealtime so that they can break the fast with a good meal while others prefer to end it at a different time of day – your choice.

Eating like this will reduce your calorie intake over the course of a week without affecting what you can eat. The only thing that is affected is how often. If you want to really succeed on this protocol though you do need to include regular workouts, especially a bit of resistance training. My sister tried this and found that although she could last for a week or so, she always lapsed back into her normal pattern and thus put on weight again, creating the yoyo effect. If you have any doubts about your ability to keep on the plan, go for the first option rather than this one because yoyo dieting isn't at all healthy.

Pros: - This protocol is highly flexible although, for some, 24 hours may seem like a long time to go without eating. In fact, to start with you don't have to go for 24 hours – go for as long as you can without eating on the first day and gradually build it up, let your body get used to not eating. Perhaps the best time to start is when you have a busy day ahead of you or you don't have any meals out planned.

Plus, there is no food that is forbidden on this method. All you have to do is exercise caution in how much you eat – for example, you can have a slice of cake, just don't eat the whole thing!

Cons: - It will be tough for some people to go 24 hours without any calorie intake and some of you will experience the usual side effects of no food – headaches, irritability, etc. These effects will disappear as time goes by, the more your body gets used to the fast. There is also the temptation to binge at the end of the fast and, although this can be stopped, it does take an awful lot of self-control, which some people simply don't have. If you are one of those people who try all kinds of diets and fails, this isn't the choice for you. It's setting yourself up for failure.

20-hour Fast

This is for those of you who like following rules and who are devoted to their cause.

How it works: For this method, you should be prepared to fast for 20 hours each day and just eat one meal every night, a fairly large one. However, the timing of your meal and what you actually eat are also important. This is based on working with the circadian rhythm of your body (that is the rhythm that dictates your body clock) and that, in actual fact, human beings are programed to eat at night.

The 20-hour fast is more about eating less than eating nothing. You can eat raw vegetables or fruit, protein and drink fresh juice if you need to. This is designed to make the most of the Sympathetic Nervous System – that determined our fight or flight response – and this promotes energy, alertness and kick-starts the fat burning process.

The reason the 4-hour main eating period is at night is so that your Parasympathetic Nervous System is prompted into maximizing your body's ability to recover and it aids digestion, relaxation and a feeling of peace. This, in turn, allows your body to put the nutrients for growth and repair to good use. Night eating also stimulates the production of hormones and fat burning during the daytime.

Day/time	Sunday	Monday	Tuesday	Weds.	Thurs.	Friday	Saturday
6-10 pm	Eating						
Sleep	Fasting						
Morning	Fasting						
Afternoon	Zero calorie						

One other important factor with this 4-hour window is the order in which you eat food groups. You should start with vegetables;

move on to protein and then fat. If you are still hungry after eating these groups (which you shouldn't be really, then you can add in some carbohydrates. I would suggest waiting for 20 minutes after finishing the third group before deciding if you are still hungry or not.

Pros: - This is seen as an easier method because you can still eat a bit during the fasting period, making it easier to get through the day. Some people also report an increase in their energy levels and the amount of fat they lose as well. It's a fairly easy routine for fast weight loss, although you may find it doesn't fit with your lifestyle.

Cons: - While it is nice to be able to eat a bit during the fast, the guidelines are strict and can be hard going for some people. The strict plan and eating guide may also interfere in any social plans that you have. And, if you are used to eating your largest meal during the day, eating one large meal at night could be difficult, especially if you find it difficult to eat late at night. I found that eating at night, even in the order shown didn't suit me at all. I suspect that I have a built in aversion to it because of my hiatus hernia problems and reflux at night, but it was too long a period to go without food and even zero calorie foods didn't make me feel that I was not being deprived. If you don't have much willpower, then this isn't a wise choice for you at all.

Combination Fast

This is ideal for those who love to workout but also like to have a cheat day every now and again.

How does it work: This is a combination of all of the above methods. You get one cheat day every week where you can eat pretty much what you want. That must be followed by a 36-hour fast though and the rest of the week is a combination of all of the above protocols.

It is best to keep your longest fast period for your busiest days. You should also continue to work out regularly, concentrating on free weights and body weight exercises, to reap the best rewards and the most fat loss. How you split the remaining fast periods is entirely up to you. I found this a bit hit and miss because it gives you too much choice and the 36-hour fast is a really hard one. I think I would rather stick to my own regime because it's easy to handle and there are no variations and no question marks.

Pros: - Technically speaking, we all fast at some point during the day, when we are not eating but, because we are not doing it at the same times every day, the results are the opposite of what we want to achieve. This plan gives you a full 7 days of fasting schedules that enable the body to get used to fasting and to get used to a timetable, thus reaping the best rewards. And, you get a full cheat day, which is a real bonus!

Cons: - The real problem comes on the cheat day, if you can't handle it in a healthy way. It is not an invitation to graze on rubbish all day long; you still have to eat in moderation and know when you have had enough. And, because the fasting periods are different each day, it can be a little bit confusing – this will be rectified with the aid of a calendar and time though. Personally, I found this gave me too much freedom and if you are a foodie like me and have a weight problem, this isn't the way to go. It gives you far too much flexibility and reason to pig out on your treat day. In fact, you automatically go for the foods that are the worst because you associate treat with something naughty.

Alternative Fasting

This is a good method for the dieter who is disciplined and has a specific goal in terms of weight.

How does it work? Possibly the easiest method of all, you can eat normally on one day, and very little on the next. On the alternative, low calorie days, you should consume no more than one-fifth of your normal calories – usually between 4-500 maximum.

To make those low days easier you can use meal replacement shakes if you want because they contain all the required nutrients and can be sipped at during the day, instead of making several meals to eat. However, these should only be used for a maximum of 14 days after which you must turn to real food on the down days. If you are a regular gym goer, try to keep your workouts to the normal days, not on the low calorie days.

Pros: - If your goal is weight loss then this is the plan for you. Cutting calories by 20-35% should achieve you a weight loss of approximately 2-2 ½ lbs. per week.

Cons: - While it is an easy one to follow, it is also very easy to be tempted into binging on your normal day of eating. Try to plan your meals ahead so you are not tempted and you don't go to an all-you-can-eat buffet hungry!

These are just 5 of the most common intermittent fasting protocols, there are many more to choose from. The real trick is experimenting, finding the one that suits you and your routine the best. If one doesn't work, move on and try another one.

Look at the charts and see which one works best with your life. Some people are much more disciplined than others. For example, the alternative fasting didn't work for me because I know that if I do that, I am effectively encouraging the yoyo effect and I saw how all of my family has gone through that effect in their lives. We were born into a family where weight gain is a known thing. We have a sweet tooth. If given the choice between a healthy carrot and a doughnut, I know exactly which choice each of us would make and this diet actually encourages you to pig out on normal days. If you have a real weight problem, the better way is to have a fast every day for a set period of time and there is no choice about what you eat on certain days and what you eat on others. You simply eat good food and there's no question of the occasional treat or binge.

It works better for me and if you are overweight, it will work better for you because it's a way of life, rather than a temporary restriction that you may not be able to keep to. As far as I am concerned, being an overweight person, anything that questions your ability to eat foods that you know are going to add to your weight problem isn't worth the risk. You know as well as I do that the temptation is too great. You give yourself the false impression that you are in control and tell yourself that the occasional treat won't hurt, but then the treats get to be more often and the purpose of the diet is lost forever.

Instead of going that route, if you come from an overweight family and you know that you are tempted by all the wrong foods, choose the option that I have where all the guidelines are clear-cut and you are less likely to cheat. One thing that I found which was very encouraging was that I feel fitter. I don't run out of breath when I walk a long way. My heart feels healthier and I know that I won't suffer from all the obesity related illnesses that my family has had to put up with all of these years. My mother yoyo dieted for over 50 years and died prematurely because of her weight. The weight that she had put a strain on her heart. You also fill up your arteries with all the wrong kind of cholesterol when you don't take care of what you eat and this is when strokes occur.

If you look after your weight and really enjoy healthy foods as much as I do, you lengthen your life expectancy and really will do yourself a favor. No diabetes, no cancer caused by over indulgence in sugar, no heart attack based on over indulgence and clogging up of arteries. Yes, of course, everyone has to die, but at least you can enjoy the life that you have and find energy right up until you are older and not have all the weight related illnesses that do turn around and bite you in your old age. My mother's life caught up with her at an early age because she didn't listen to all of the warnings. I am choosing to listen and the fasting regime that I use to help me really does make me feel healthier, gives my body more time to heal itself and helps my digestive system to eliminate toxins which would otherwise have stayed in my body for days.

I used to be permanently constipated. I used to take laxatives because it was the only way I had to be regular. What this was doing was putting a strain on my liver and kidneys because these products are not gentle. They do work, but eventually they make your bowels lazy and that's not a good option. Fasting is a great option and I can't stress enough the amount of change I have seen in the way I am able to live my life because of the choice that I made to fast every day in order to let my body process things in a much more effective way.

When you make that choice, you say goodbye to all the aches and pains. My ankles don't swell. My circulation is good. My cholesterol levels are wonderful and I don't have all of the health issues that I had before I started the fast. Would I ever go back to normal eating? To me, this way of life is normal eating. It's a lifestyle that I have adopted and is part of the way that I have chosen to live my life. I still love food and I guess I am fortunate to be a lover of all kinds of vegetables. I feed myself sufficiently with a variety of vegetables that really docs lift my spirit and make me feel like all my nutritional needs are being met.

Can you do it? Of course you can, and even if you are a foodie like me, start to learn about all the foods that you may have missed out on. I love green beans with a little dressing. I don't pig out on calorific dressings any more but I taste the food more. If you ever thought that food tastes nicer when it's cooked by someone else, find out why because you can make healthy food so enjoyable and if you decide to have second helpings, you really won't be doing your weight or your muscles any harm whatsoever.

I find that the choices available to you offer you a lot of scope but that you need to choose the one that suits your life best. The 16-hour fasting daily is potentially the easiest unless you are someone who enjoys going out in the evenings and then you may find that it's a little restrictive.

What I liked about the 16 hour fast is it's simple, it's straightforward and there's no variance every day to accommodate. My sister chose a system whereby she deprived herself of food for 24 hours at a time and it was harder. She did lose weight, but she didn't keep that weight off because of course, you can't sustain this over a long period of time without feeling that it's doing something it shouldn't do. 24 hours is a long time between one meal and another, so I chose to opt for something more predictable and sustaining so that I would be able to keep it up even after having lost the weight that I wanted to lose. Incidentally, I went down two sizes and I think that my body has stabilized now at a specific weight that I am happy with.

Since I don't want to go back to being fat, I am not prepared to change my lifestyle again. As stated earlier, the easier you make your diet, the more likely you are to keep to it. Yoyo diets, where you deprive yourself of certain foods and then reintroduce them when you have achieved weight loss are a bad idea. You put your body through so much confusion and end up fatter than when you started so avoid the yoyo. Go for a way of life and decide based upon your own lifestyle which fasting suits you the best and which you can sustain over a long period of time. I won't go back on my fasting because I can see what a difference it has made to the way that I think and process thoughts as well as to the way my muscles are toned and slim and my body is able to digest food. After a lifetime of constipation, that was a miracle and it's one worthwhile holding onto. No more bloat and no more embarrassing moments, as well as there being no need at all to take laxatives which eventually do damage the system and make it even lazier than it used to be.

Fasting is easy. There is no calorie counting. There is no need to weigh out your food or go to extremes when it comes to choosing what's nutritious and good for you. Common sense tells you that. You don't need to measure what you eat. You just need to be savvy about what your body is capable of eating and whether that amount of food is helping you to shape up or not. If it's not, up the ante and cut out some of the foods you know contain carbs and sugar. It's really as simple as that.

Brian Adams

Top Tricks and Tips for Intermittent Fasting

You might be thinking, at this stage, that this is going to be difficult. The first tip I have for you is to stop thinking that. The more you think it will be difficult, the more it will be; it is as simple as that. When I chose the fasting routine that I chose, I did so because it was the most natural for me. I didn't like breakfast anyway and the only alteration I had to make in the mornings was drinking black coffee without sugar instead of white coffee with sweeteners. I thought that if I was going to go this far, then the sweeteners could go as well because they simply boost your sugar levels for a short time and then make you crave more. It is actually easier on the head to give up all sugar during the fast period and forget about it. I used this period for drinking more water. I knew that I didn't drink enough water to start off with and this gave me the incentive I needed to push my water levels up. That's a positive move and made all my skin problems go away and that's a big thing for me, since my skin had been terrible for years.

Doctors had told me about drinking water for years but it had fallen on deaf ears. We don't hear what we don't want to hear. I had experienced muscle problems for as long as I could remember and I also remember an osteopath telling me that if I drank water regularly, then I wouldn't have the muscle spasms that I was experiencing and he was right. I hate to admit it but that was also the cause of constipation to a certain level and all the water that I am now drinking instead of coffee and tea mean that my body is detoxing daily. That's got to be a good thing. I don't suffer from wind after I eat any more and I feel great.

Stop freaking about it - Stop asking yourself if it will harm you to just fast for 15 hours instead of 16 or if eating an apple on your fasting period is bad for you. Relax and get into it, give your body a chance to adapt to your new lifestyle. I don't cheat at all because I know that if I did, I would be cheating myself. It is this type of unwarranted fear that makes many a person nervous and they decide to not take the diet seriously. But the whole point is for you to take it up seriously and ensure that you develop and maintain a fit body. But don't assume your body will not put up a fight. It is obvious that you will feel like giving up on it all too easy but that is not the way forward. You have to make up your mind to stick with the diet and not freak out about its various small aspects.

It's not all cut and dried – if you don't feel like eating breakfast one day but you do the next then that's fine. You only need to be rigid in your discipline if you are going for peak athletic fitness. Stop stressing, it will just make you more tempted to eat what you shouldn't, when you shouldn't. In my case, what I found was that I fell into the routine fairly easily. My partner, on the other hand, tended to keep making me coffee with milk and sugar for a while, but he soon got the hang of it. We socialize during the hours that I am permitted to eat and rarely go out for an evening meal, so it suited me fine that I couldn't eat after 8 at night. That was a no brainer and it stopped the snacks in front of the TV. Instead of snacking, I found myself drinking a glass of water and being satisfied with all the food that I had eaten during the day.

Expect people to look at you in a funny way. It will happen, when you tell someone you no longer eat breakfast or don't eat for a whole day. Don't even bother trying to explain it because most people simply won't understand what you are doing or why. Just get on with your way of life and fit it in around your schedule. In this way, I didn't actually have anyone question me about my choices because no one ever saw me at breakfast time anyway and as I said, my socializing was always at lunchtime rather than in the evening, so I didn't stress about having to tell people my routine. If you are worried about it fitting with your lifestyle, choose the option that I did because it really is the easiest to work into your day without any problem at all. I don't even pig out at 7.30 in the evening in preparation any more as I used to when I first started. Now, I just let the day pass and eat at times that are suitable to me, rather than think that the kitchen is going to be closed in half an hour. You need to get your head around it in a very positive way. I lost so much weight but it did take effort and it took incorporating exercise into my daily routine. That's not hard when you make it fun.

Keep busy

Don't spend long period sitting around because you'll start to think about how hungry you are and you'll be more likely to struggle and cave in. Try to time your fasting periods for the maximum benefit:

Start just after a huge meal – you'll be so stuffed you won't even think about eating. I didn't do this but it works for some people. Plan your fast to take place overnight – that's a good 6-8 hours of it gone already.

Keep busy. That'll take care of a few hours of the fast and it will go quicker than you thought it would. Don't indulge in thinking about your diet. Let it do its job and you do yours. Don't keep thinking about it and wasting your time. Concentrate on other things around you.

It's okay to drink calorie free beverages. Try green tea in the mornings, which will give you a caffeine kick. Drink plenty of water and stay hydrated. This is important – hunger is often mistaken for thirst so aim for at least 2-4 liters of plain water a day – add a slice of lemon if you want a kick. You can drink black coffee as well; just don't add sugar or milk.

Listen to your body. It will tell you all you need to know. Monitor your training, keep an eye on your body fat, and track what you eat and your calorie consumption. Watch how your body changes when you eat the same amount of calories but change when you eat and how you eat them.

No two people will react to the method of eating the same way so it's important that you monitor your own body signs.

Don't expect overnight miracles, it won't happen. Many diets and fasts out there promise you such things but they are only lying to you. Intermittent fasting will help you to lose weight and it will increase your sensitivity to insulin and your growth hormone production. But, this is only one small part of determining your health and composition so don't expect to lose loads of weight instantly just by missing a meal. Focus on eating healthily, better foods and on increasing your strength. My muscles feel wonderfully supple. They used to feel rock hard. I know that my body is thanking me for caring sufficiently to make it a lean mean machine!

Stress and weight gain

As you know, stress is responsible for many problems in life. You may think that stress only affects those that lead stressful lives and have a big work responsibility. But that is not true. Stress can affect any one and any time and any situation can bring it on. You must know how to combat stress and remain as calm and positive as possible. In this chapter, we will look at the correlation between stress and weight gain and why it is important for you to keep your stress to a bare minimum while you are on the intermittent fast.

Stress has a direct connection with weight gain. The human mind controls the entire body and it's functioning. When a person stresses out he or she has an over load of cortisol secreted in their brain!

This can affect their everyday life and make it impossible for them to operate optimally on a daily basis. Although cortisol is said to be a good chemical as it allows the person to operate optimally, it can cause them to have limited movement.

This can lead to the person feeling tired and fatigued and having no enthusiasm to carry out the different important mundane routines. When that happens, the body goes into an over drive to help the brain function optimally. When that happens, the rest of the body does not know what to do. So you end up doing all the wrong things and affect your body in a negative way.

Right from consuming junk foods to cutting down on sleep, you end up doing all things you must not do. In that, these things will only negate your diet and cause you to remain regretful. Stress will also make it impossible for you to stick with your fast and you will keep breaking the rules every so often without caring about the consequences.

So the need of the hour is to combat stress as much as possible and not allow it to affect your intermittent fast.

I know it sounds impossible but it is compulsory for you to combat your stress and not allow it to affect your fast in any which way.

So to start with, address all the stressors in your life and make sure you sort everything out at the earliest. For most people, work and family is what causes stress and you must address all issues related to these at the earliest. The basic intention is to fix the problems that give you tension and root it out if possible.

The first step is to make a list of all the stressors and write it down neatly. Next, address it one by one and ensure that it does not bother you again. Regardless of whether it is related to your finances or your personal life, sort everything out and eliminate the stress from your life.

But whatever you do, you can of course not eliminate stress 100% and must make efforts to reduce it to a bare minimum. For this, here are certain things that you can do to cut down on stress.

The very first thing to do is create time for yourself. In this day and age where everything is fast paced, people tend to forget about themselves and how important it is to put one's own needs first. Stop neglecting yourself and take time out to pamper yourself. Take a few days off and take a vacation. Just ensure that you continue with the intermittent fast on your vacation as well. Take a partner along and the two of you can remain motivated to stop stressing out and consuming healthy nutritious food.

Next, modify your lifestyle. Cut down on indulging in activities that promote stress. This can include attending meetings where you feel stressed or doing something guilty. If you have a bad habit then consider kicking it. You must remain true to yourself and do things that are good for you and your body.

Next up, indulge in some meditation. Meditation is a great way to relax the mind and get rid of unnecessary stress. You must focus on increasing the control that you have over your mind and doing things that do not affect you negatively. Find a quiet corner in your house and start chanting a calming word. Continue doing so until you feel tired. This will completely eliminate your stress in no time and you can return to your normal life once again.

Take up a hobby that you enjoy. Indulging in it will distract you from stress and also the diet. It can be singing, dancing, painting or cooking. As long as it diverts your attention, you can take it up and exploit it. Enjoy yourself and don't allow tiny upheavals to affect you negatively.

Avoid negative people. There can be many people out there determined to make you look and feel bad. This can include colleagues and other such people. If someone is making fun of your fast then ignore them. Remember that you are doing it for yourself and to attain and maintain a fit and healthy body. Other people's opinions should not matter much and you must remain as optimistic as possible.

Lastly, try to enjoy your fasting journey. Don't allow it to stress you out and remain as motivated and rooted as possible. Don't stop with it even after achieving your health goal and continue pursuing it until you feel like it has transformed into a lifestyle change.

These are just some of the things that you can do to combat your stress and it is important that you put in efforts to consciously keep stress out of your life. It will be easier said than done but since you know how bad stress can really be, you must make the effort to kick it out of your life permanently.

The Health Benefits of Fasting

Although we have briefly mentioned health benefits in previous chapters, the reason why I think it's important to point this out in a chapter of its own is because fasting is life changing. It doesn't just improve your lifestyle, but it can actually help you to live for a longer period of time.

As was mentioned in the history of fasting segment, the various beneficial effects of fasting have been known to man for hundreds of years. There was a reason why mankind decided to take up fasting and that reason was to explore the different health benefits that fasting actually provided. Till now, I'm sure you know of generic benefits that fasting provides to those who take it up and now, we will look at specific benefits.

Let's start to look at ways in which this helps. The biggest hurdle that people have to jump over when they are looking at their health and nutrition is that temptation to binge or to eat between meals. Because fasting effectively starves your body of all the bad things during the fast period, it also gives the body more time to deal with the things that you did eat. You may think that binging when you are permitted is the way that it will end up, but what happens is the opposite. You lose the taste for snacks because it feels so good losing the fat from your body and you actually lose the taste for sweet snacks. Cut out all the bad fats and you are still left with a wonderful variety of food to eat and you don't even need to use sweeteners.

I found out a long time ago that sweeteners are actually sweeter than sugar and that your body craves that extra sugar when you don't have your sweeteners around. Natural sugar from fruits lasts much longer and gives you a better buzz than any sweetener can. Thus, I was able to kick the sweeteners and although I do love the occasion sweet taste, I found that I was more drawn toward healthy alternatives. Instead of ice cream, I took to eating sorbet which is water based instead of being milk based. Instead of using the wrong oils and butter, I changed to using Omega 3 spread and Olive oil.

Cancer

If you have never had cancer, talk to someone who has. Interestingly enough, they test you by making you eat sugar because the cancers in your body are drawn toward it. That's got to tell you that sugar encourages cancer. Thus, if you are able to cut down on all the sugared items during your fast – and I did and I was a sugar freak – you are cutting down your risks of attracting cancer or making it spread to other places in the body if it does happen.

Heart disease

It's obvious that if you replace bad fats with good ones, you free up your arteries and don't prolong the clogging effect that bad foods have. If your arteries are clogged, you can't breathe properly and you lose breath when you exert yourself. You can't function because your heart stops you from doing all the things that you want to do. You are more prone to swollen ankles and if you eat all the wrong foods are likely to have high levels of cholesterol, which can spell heart attack or stroke. There's no question about this at all. Since being on the fast, I am able to walk longer distances. I am able also to enjoy an occasional treat and not feel bad about it because I know that I give my body sufficient time to process all the foods that I have eaten during the time that I am permitted to eat.

Obesity

What this basically means is that your body fat mass is too great for your size. You are fat. This can be caused by a variety of things, but when you deal with it by having an intermittent fast, you also help your body to use up the excess fat that you may have accumulated and to get yourself back on track. If, on the other hand, you decide not to do anything about it, you can find yourself getting diabetes, which is for life. You also need to know that your heart, your liver, your kidneys, your circulation and everything within your body needs a free flow. If you are fat, you don't give your body the chance to maximize on health being good. In fact, if you know yourself to be obese, as I did, you have a responsibility to yourself to actually do something positive toward losing that weight. Strokes, heart attacks and all kinds of illnesses can attack people who are obese because they don't have the same resistance to illness that other people have.

The other thing is that you don't have the same mobility. If you have ever felt puffed out when you did the slightest exercise, then chances are you need to do something. If you don't, things won't improve. I knew this and I also knew my family history and knew that if I didn't do something, I could end up in an early grave and it seemed a little silly not to do something while I still had the choice.

Mental clarity

When you undertake this fast, your mind and body will both benefit from it. The diet will make you sharper and increase your memory. So you will remember things better and can use it to your advantage. In fact, you can also take advantage of the situation and improve your cognition as well. Join a book club or a reading club and exercise your brain's cells. You can also join a language class and increase your thinking power.

Glowing skin

The intermittent fast is a diet that helps in eliminating toxins from the body. These toxins are capable of causing internal damage, which can show up on the skin. So it is important that you follow the diet carefully. The intake of excess water helps remove tiredness and your skin will develop a unique glow. Apart from the internal intake, you must also do a few external beauty regimes, which will help you further enhance the effects. Simple things like washing your face with mild detergents and applying an external pack made from fresh fruits will further add to your beauty.

Shiny mane

Who does not wish to have shiny hair? When you take up this diet, your hair will turn quite shiny. All you have to do is follow a strict intermittent fast and you will see the results in no time. Water helps in eliminating build up and also flushes out other toxins that might be causing your scalp to turn oily. The intake of fresh fruits and vegetables further adds to your hair's quality. By including foods rich in proteins, you will be enhancing your hair's capacity to develop strength and improve their tensile quality.

Stronger teeth

Your teeth will also strengthen when you take up the diet. You must, however, follow the diet strictly. You need strong teeth for life. Given the amount of junk foods and sodas that you consume, your teeth will start to corrode in no time. So it is best that you take up this diet and say good-bye to all your unhealthy eating habits. You will feel completely rejuvenated and happy after taking up the diet and wish to continue with it for a long time.

Autophagy

Autophagy refers to the cells in your body fixing themselves up. So they will remove all the unwanted toxic waste and help your cells grow strong. The foods that you eat will be full of anti-oxidants and you can easily increase your immunity as well. As you've already seen, the diet helps combat several illnesses and promotes good health.

Growth hormones

As people age, the growth hormones start to get affected. So it is important that you help your body remain fit for long and encourage it to secrete growth hormones. This is possible if you maintain a strict intermittent diet. The diet will help your cells remain strong and healthy for long and in turn, increase your body's capacity to produce the different growth hormones.

You only get one shot at this life. If you don't take it seriously, you really will suffer in the long term and you may be too late to actually make things right. By going onto the intermittent fast, you are saying "no" to the kind of bad health that is associated with so many people in this day and age and "yes!" to life. It's as simple as that. The fast will improve your health. It will reverse certain health issues but don't leave it until it's too late to put things into reverse. Giving up on the idea of healthy diet is stupidity and will certainly lead you to a death, which comes before your time. Take a look at people around you. There is so much obesity that it is becoming a real nightmare from a healthcare point of view. You never know, your kids may even see what you are doing and join you in your fasting. I would never advise it during the growing period, but when a child is obese and has problems breathing, it's a better alternative than the lifestyle that he/she has.

Brian Adams

Deciding on the Start of Your Fast

Now that you have all the details, it's up to you to decide which type of fast you want to go on. Each has its pros and cons and it's really down to lifestyle and which you believe you can fit in with your lifestyle. You need to do a little preparation. You need to get rid of foods that you know are not good for you. The replacements shown below are good solid replacements that will make your life much healthier.

Substitute foods

- Substitute white bread with whole grain bread; if this is not available then you can make some yourself. Learn to make it and have a spare loaf available at all times

- Substitute butter with Omega3 based spread, you can try sprinkling some flax seeds into your bread so that supplementary omega 3 is added into your diet

- Substitute full cream milk with skimmed milk or half cream, again, you can make this yourself, just boil the milk and wait for it to cool down, remove the thick layer of cream that forms on top and discard it, your skimmed milk is now ready to consume

- Replace white sugar with brown sugar, if you have the capacity then do away with sugar altogether

- Replace coffee with decaffeinated coffee, you can buy yourself a coffee maker and prepare it in advance to save on time and effort

- Replace starch laden vegetables for more healthy alternatives, make a list of all the best ones to savor and get them in bulk, this will ensure that you carefully pick the vegetables and don't go about it in a disorganized manner

- Get rid of red meat altogether, if you are too used to it then make a slow transition, stock up on white meat that is skinned and start replacing the red meats in your regular meals one by one

These may sound a little harsh. You can get by without changing your foods but you don't speed up the process by sticking with the same foods and these may lead you back into bad habits.

Apart from doing these things, there are certain coking tips that you can make use of to make it easier for yourself.

Start by buying yourself a slow cooker. Also known as a crock-pot, these are meant to make it easier for you to cook your food. As you know, a diet will mean changing up your meal schedule. But the intermittent diet is slightly flexible provided you remain within the boundaries of the diet.

So cooking food can be made easy and fun by placing all your ingredients in the crock-pot. It will slowly cook the vegetables and meats and you can choose a time ranging between 4 hours to 8 hours. So as soon as you wake up in the morning, add in all the ingredients and close the crock-pot. Wait for it to cook and for around 6 hours and have your first meal. Then, place fresh ingredients again and have your food ready by your dinnertime. Repeat every day until a habit forms. The nutrition will remain locked in the crock-pot.

If you don't have the patience for it then consider buying yourself a pressure cooker, which will do the opposite of a crock pot. You will have your meals ready in no time, as the cooker will take only a few minutes to cook for you. The nutrition will remain locked in the ingredients and you will have a meal ready in no time at all.

Apart from this, you must plan your entire week's meal in advance. Knowing what you will be eating will make it easier to cook your meals. Draw up a plan and mention the meals that will work well for your body. It is important to introduce variety otherwise you will start getting bored of your foods. Don't repeat the same meal two days in a row and try to incorporate rare flavors.

You can also save some food for the next day by placing it in boxes and stocking them into the fridge. This will ensure that you have a ready meal and can heat it and consume it. It might actually be extremely important for you to do this if you are a working professional and don't have the time to cook after a tiring day's work.

Plan your exercise routine

If you plan your sports activities you are more likely to stick with them. For example, tennis is something you can fix up with a friend. If you want to do dancing like I do, get yourself a video. I watch this on my iPad and it's super quality and is only a YouTube video so you don't need to spend out. Type Zumba into the search in YouTube and keep the video to favorites.

Try to replace driving as much as possible with walking. Try to take the stairs instead of taking the escalator.

Your sports activity is again up to you, but if you really want to see your body change shape and get healthy, even small changes make all the difference in the world.

These exercises are extremely important and you will read in a future chapter how you can exercise on a regular basis and the different forms of exercise that will target one specific muscle in your body at a time. You will realize that exercise is sculpting your body and your diet is helping you remain energetic all throughout your workout.

Be prepared for the wait

When you fast, it takes a couple of weeks before you start to feel differently about your life. Then you start to burn body fat as part of your body's routine and that's when you start to feel really good about what you are doing. Be prepared for this wait and be patient with yourself because it's well worth it. This isn't a short-term commitment. It's a long term one and it's going to change your life forever. But don't worry if you are actually seeing faster results. Many people's body will have a lot of puppy fat that is easy to get rid of. You will wonder how you ended up losing so much weight without having to put in lot of effort. The truth of the matter remains that your body will definitely see a change provided you know how to work it. But patience will come in handy and you have to be willing to wait for a month or two to see the results. It is general belief that what you do this month will only show the next month and the results are always cumulative in nature.

Print out your plan

Now that you have the plan, take a couple of copies so that you can put them in the kitchen area, on the fridge and can even have one with you in the evenings to remind you of your deadline. Try not to think of these as deadlines. Try to think of them as normal processes during the course of your life, like getting up, going to the bathroom, washing your hair, taking a shower. The problem with making it a deadline is that you tend to psychologically need something to eat at five minutes to eight, knowing that you have to stop eating at eight, when normally you wouldn't even bother eating at this time anyway. If you can think of it as a normal part of your day, it's a healthier attitude to have. It is believed that speaking about your plans on social media platforms or telling others about it goes a long way in helping you remain motivated and increasing your chances of tuning the diet into a success. But you have to remain positive and not allow any negative comment or remark upset you. Society will be interested in brining someone down but you have to remain strong and positive no matter what and ensure that you care about your body just as much you care about anything else.

Discuss with friends and family

This isn't obligatory but if you think that it will alter your social life, it's best to tell people in advance that you will be available for meals at midday but not in the evening. By letting people know and enthusing about your reasons, you are actually reinforcing your belief that it will work. You are also giving them the reasons why and if they care about you, they will respect your limitations and not offer you food at times when you are not permitted to eat under your new lifestyle regime. This might be especially important if you are extremely social or have a big family that keeps meeting all the time. You might have to implement a no forcing me rule and make it clear to everyone that you are not interested in breaking your diet habit whatsoever. If you do feel pressured then tell them that you will only do whatever is comfortable for you. But no friends and family will actually try to stand in your way and you can find your strength in them. I found that friends actually noticed the difference and asked me what my secret was! When I mentioned fasting, they had forgotten about that because it had been so long ago that I started that no one really noticed any more.

Brian Adams

Things That Will Deter Weight Loss and Muscle Formation

If you are really serious about looking after your health interests, you do need to incorporate some kind of exercise and regular drinking of water. Don't be lulled into thinking that drinking coffee or tea is drinking water. The difference between coffee and tea and actually drinking water is a lot. Tea and coffee are stimulants and they tend to make you urinate more often. I remember an osteopath telling me this and I never forgot it. If you drink one cup of coffee, you urinate three. That means that your body is losing water content. The consequences of this are dehydration, tiredness, and muscle weakness and skin conditions.

If you drink water, you will therefore feel less tired, and more capable of exercising and thus are much more likely to last. You may wonder if you always need exercise in your life but the answer to this one is common sense. The body needs to move to keep its strength and to firm up muscles. Thus, the answer is affirmative. A certain amount of exercise is necessary in everyone's life and that includes those who have illnesses that stop him or her from full physical exercise. For those people who are bedridden, for example, a physiotherapist may suggest leg lifts or arm exercises to help the body to regain its strength. I know in the case of my father, we had to supervise exercises of his legs where we had to place a certain weight on them and he was then expected to lift and lower the legs. It doesn't matter what state of health you are in, you need a certain amount of exercise and it's vital to good health.

Getting a dog may encourage elderly people who are not accustomed to exercise. The dog will always need walking and if that's all the exercise that they get, it's better than nothing at all. If you find yourself limited in any way, look for alternative style exercises because these are every bit as valid for firming up muscle. I had a period with a slipped disc where movement was almost impossible, though I still managed to do exercises which didn't affect the back too badly at all.

Lack of exercise will deter muscle strengthening and weight loss. Thus, include it as part of your daily life because it's essential.

Unhealthy food choices

The food that you choose to eat will make a difference to weight loss. You do need a varied diet that avoids obvious pitfalls such as carbohydrates. Does this mean I never eat doughnuts? No, it doesn't, but it does mean that I know the price I have to pay if I make that choice. What I tend to do is make myself go without something when I am presented with tempting food when visiting or when I am simply tempted myself to have something I know not to be the best for me. Since this is a lifestyle change, I can't deprive myself of the occasional treat, but I can make a bargain with myself occasionally that allows me that luxury. For example, if you have that doughnut, you can cut back on dressings on the salad. That's not a big hardship. If I have a slice of white bread, I can make sure that I cut something down later.

I don't calorie count, but I do keep an eye on what I eat and know when I need to forfeit something because I have been over indulgent. As long as you have a common sense feel for what you eat, it's okay to be naughty occasionally. Just don't let all the bad foods creep back into your larder.

Cutting out sleep

Never think that you can cut out your sleep. It's part of your treatment. It's part of your lifestyle and it's essential to healing and to processing the foods that you have eaten during the course of the day. You may not know this but people who deprive themselves of sleep are not more productive. They may be awake for more hours, but their minds become sluggish because the body and mind need sleep. If this is an area of neglect in your life it can stem your weight loss. You may not be aware of it, but during the sleep process, your body is burning up calories in the healing process that a human body goes through during the hours of sleep.

If you find that it's hard to get off to sleep, evaluate why. Perhaps you have your computer in your bedroom and allow it to take precedence over sleep. I have one friend that blamed a sleep disorder when in fact, he was someone who lived alone and didn't do all of the daily chores that people do because he had no routine to life. He used to stay up late at night on the computer and go to bed at about three or four and then wonder why he couldn't get up in the mornings, blaming it on a sleep ailment when in fact it was his lack of routine within his life that led him to being unable to sleep.

In the next chapter you will look at a few tips to increase your sleep!

Increasing your sleep time

Now it is given that you will not be able to sleep longer and better just by thinking it. You will have to do things for it to happen and so, here are some useful tips on how you can sleep better and increase your diet's potency.

Chamomile

The first thing to do is consume chamomile tea. Chamomile tea is made from dried chamomile flowers that are powdered and added to tea bags. You can sip on this tea just before hitting the bed and you will not be disappointed with the results. But ensure that you buy only trusted and branded tea bags and not some duplicates. If you are not a tea drinker then you can add a little turmeric powder to a glass of warm milk and consume before retiring. This blend will surely help you sleep much better. But try to drink at least an hour before retiring and choose skim milk.

Music

Music is a great relaxant and will help you sleep better. Ensure that the music you choose is soothing and melodious. Avoid loud music and contemporary songs. You can also choose classical songs and compositions, which are actually meant to put you to sleep. Your mind will feel relaxed and you won't have to worry about the various stressors. Have the music on auto play and attach a timer to it so that you won't have to get up in the middle of the night to put in into play or stop it. Natural sounds such as the sound of water falls and jungle sounds will also help you sleep better and increase your body's capacity to heal while you sleep.

Lighting

Making use of mood lighting is a great way to increase your sleep time. Although it is recommended that you sleep in a fully dark room where there is only 2% light, this can be mood lighting. Choose colors that are soothing to you like light green or light purple. By focusing on a dim light, you will not only feel sleepy but also gain restful sleep. You can have the light directly above you or at a short distance. Don't focus too much on the light though and try and maintain peripheral vision.

Aroma

Natural scents also have the capacity to improve your sleep. You have to burn something natural like sage leaves or Vetiver and place it under the bed. You can also choose something more aromatic like rose petals or burn aromatherapy candles. Spraying something natural and aromatic on your sheets or in your bedroom will also work wonders. But ensure that it is all natural and there are no chemicals in it. The best scents to try out include rose, sandal, bay leaves, cinnamon and jasmine. If you don't want a strong odor then consider placing a couple of jasmine flowers under your pillow. But change them every day.

Media

One thing that most people do before retiring to bed is either watch television or partake in social media activities! Both of these, however, are extremely potent in making you stay up at night. The visuals that these provide to you will keep roaming in your head and not allow you to have restful sleep. So try to avoid watching television as much as possible and also avoid going to bed with your cellphone. If you are already used to doing these then try to reduce it slowly. Going too fast might cause you to have a relapse so don't go about it the wrong way.

Partner

Getting a partner to remind you to hit the bed early and keep telling you about its benefits will help you sleep faster and longer. Also, you must avoid having unnecessary tiffs with your loved ones and remain as peaceful as possible when you go to sleep. Many times, saying a simple thank you to your loved ones will make you feel lighter and give you the chance to sleep better. So try to do that every now and then and then hit the bed, as it will help you sleep better.

Work

Don't carry your work tensions to bed. You will not feel like sleeping at all. So stop thinking about work at least an hour before bed. That will not only help you relax but also increase your enthusiasm to sleep and provide your mind with some relaxation. If you do carry your tensions to bed, try to shift focus to something else like reading an interesting book before retiring. Do everything in your power to relax as much as possible before hitting the bed.

Massage

Going in for a relaxing massage before hitting the bed is always a good idea! You can either visit a massage parlor or invite a masseuse home. It will also be a good idea to ask your spouse to give you a massage. A warm oil massage will be best and you can use aromatic oil like sandal. You can look up online videos that instruct you to massage the right way. Make sure you don't over do it and try to press the right pressure points on your body.

Exercise

Although exercising is a great activity to take up to beat stress effectively, it is best to avoid exercising close to bedtime. If you exercise too much, then you will end up feeling over excited. So if you plan to exercise in the evening, then ensure that you stop at least 2 hours before bedtime. Remain relaxed and only then go to bed.

Apart from these, you can also meditate a little and then go to sleep, as that will help you remain relaxed. You can also download an app that records your sleep activity and tell you the times when you slept well and when you dint. Try to capitalize on the sleep pattern and increase your deep sleep.

Get a routine. Make your life much more enjoyable by keeping to it and you will find that your body will really feel much livelier and that your weight will simply disappear, even while you are sleeping.

Brian Adams

Medications and Potential Side Effects

When you take up a diet for the first time, it is obvious that your body will take time to adjust. However, you must ensure that you are the right candidate for the diet and you have the capacity to withstand it. For that, you must do some research and know whether it is safe for you to carry out the diet. You cannot take your health for granted and must ensure that your body will not face any negative consequences.

Usually, if you have medications to take, you take these at a set time. Some may need to be taken at mealtimes. If this were the case, then you would be better opting for the choice that I made of a 16 hour fast every day. That way, you can still take your medications at lunchtime and they won't affect you in an adverse way.

The medications that are particularly bad to take without food really should be taken with meals, so you may need to time fasting periods according to what your medical needs are. For example, anti-inflammatory medications may give you stomach problems if not taken at mealtimes and so may antibiotics. Ask your doctor first before taking up any diet and ensure that he or she writes you a plan to follow. Many people assume things and end up doing wrong things. If you rely on assumptions then you might put your body through unnecessary trauma. So be sure first and only then take the next step.

If you are in doubt about any of your regular meds, talk to your doctor immediately and discuss what you are about to do, so that a time can be sorted out to take your medications regularly without upsetting your body's routine. If the doctor is unavailable then wait for him and then take up after a consultation. Until such time, don't think it will be okay to do things by yourself.

If you are diabetic or have pre-existing illnesses, do talk to your general practitioner before you start the fast. My doctor was quite agreeable about it because he could see that weight loss would actually improve any health problems that I had. In fact, he encouraged it. But that can vary from person to person and you must know for sure whether or not something will work for you. If you still have doubts about it then it is best to go in for a complete body analysis to understand whether or not it is safe to take up the diet and improve your overall health.

The quality of life that you have can be improved by fasting, as has been shown in studies that were done on people who were suffering from asthma and who were overweight. What the studies proved was that our survival instincts kick in when we fast and it makes the body much more likely to respond by taking fat from the body to survive and that's exactly what you want it to do.

You must understand that this diet is not designed only for men and is suitable for women as well. Those suffering from illnesses owing to obesity will find this diet extremely helpful. The main goal is to cut out the fat and increase the nutrition that the body gets. This is possible by formulating a good diet plan and more importantly, sticking with it. If you think it is not possible for you to follow the diet then take it slow. Rushing into something will often cause it to come undone. So don't be in a hurry and take it one day at a time if you wish the results to stick for a longer time.

If you are pregnant or nursing then it is best to take the doctor's advice first. He might suggest a modification. The same extends to children and old people as there will be many things to consider before taking up a diet and it is important to consult the doctor fast to remain on the safer side.

Thus, it's very unlikely that you will find problems arising if you take your fasting seriously and follow a good healthy diet. One should always remember that the food that we eat determines the kind of lifestyle we end up having, but that fasting helps the process by giving the body a well-needed break. If you do take meds, make sure that you can do this with your meals and if morning pills are taken, you can always take them with a glass of water. If in doubt, consult your doctor.

My Experience at Intermittent Fasting

I felt quite hyped up about the idea as soon as I heard about it because it fit with my lifestyle. I didn't like eating in the mornings anyway so it wasn't a hardship to give up morning food. The hardest task was going to be stopping my partner from offering me snacks during the course of the evening, and with this in mind, I told my partner to resist the temptation. After all, my health came first.

I liked the fact that everything was so clear cut and easy. For example, I didn't have to worry too much about what I was preparing for myself in the way of food, because as long as I was sensible and kept off bad fats, I would lose fat. I also liked the fact that I wasn't actually restricting my intake during the hours that I was permitted to eat. Did I ever feel like cheating? Not really, but I did start to get the panics when it came to close to eight in the evening, but soon realized that it was silly. It's like people drinking five pints of beer fast just because the pub is about to close. That mentality has never been mine, so associating the dilemma with that mentality put a stop to it.

Drinking water was never something I did enough of. The osteopath was right. Had I drunk water on a regular basis in the past, I may have saved myself a lot of inflammation and tired muscle. I don't have that problem now so I know that it's associated with drinking water. I actually got to the stage of not really noticing what I was drinking early on in the fast and have never looked back. I used to drink black coffee and then said that instead of that, I could replace it with water and cut coffee back to after my main meal. Coffee isn't that good for you anyway and at least that way I still got one cup of coffee a day which was warm and welcomed.

In the first week, I guess I noticed a little that I missed the snacks, but that deprivation didn't seem to go on for that long because it's just like changing a routine. Once the new routine has set in, you don't really question it. I sleep more these days than I did before and I always used to stay up late working and managed to stop that habit in its tracks. If you are going to go without food for 16 hours, then you need your full night of sleep and although I never thought I needed that much sleep am actually glad that I decided to conform because it makes the hours of fasting go faster and thus I don't really miss the food that I ate during those hours which had now become fasting hours.

I did an experiment and wrote down what I missed the most, and these will likely figure in your calculations as well.

- White bread

- Cakes

- Biscuits

- Crisps

- Potatoes

- Red meat

- Sauces

These were things that my body had become accustomed to eating and the first week was probably the hardest week. I was brought up to have potatoes at every meal so it was a little strange cutting back on the starch, but I am glad I did. Cakes and biscuits were fill-ins during the evening while we were watching TV and were not really that important. Instead of eating these, I found ways to keep myself busy so that I would not miss them. Yes, we walk past a cake shop occasionally and I am tempted, but only during eating time and then only if I am prepared to go without something and pay some kind of penalty. The kinds of penalties that you can give yourself are sensible things such as:

- Disallow something else with high calories

- Exercise more to make up for what it was you ate

It's common sense and second nature after a while and I don't feel that the fasting has done my body any harm at all. Now, my waistline is slimmer, my stomach is flatter and I have muscles that don't hurt any more. Contributing factors are indeed water and the intermittent fasting. Water is a real boost and since I have been drinking it I have had no real muscle problems and much better skin so it's a win-win situation. Do I enjoy the fasting? The truth is I don't really think about it anymore. Food was never my priority in life. I just let myself have things that I should have been more restrictive with. Now I can practically eat whatever I want and as long as I compensate for it, I don't suffer from weight gain and I don't feel bad about it.

What to Expect When You Start Your Fast

I think that I expected everything to happen much quicker than it actually did. I was boasting to my sister about fasting and she wasn't seeing any difference in my figure. That was until about the third week. By this time, I guess the body had used up all the excess sugar and carbs and was burning into the fat that I had accumulated over a long period of time. You won't lose weight overnight. Your muscles won't tighten overnight, but when all of those good things happen, you get a really good sense of wellbeing that you may not have felt for years.

We go through our lives not really looking at consequence. My bulky waistline was the consequence of a life spent not really taking responsibility for my body. You will begin to feel it when the body starts to feed on fat. I remember waking up one day and going to try on a pair of pants that hadn't fit for a while and finding that they were actually loose! The feeling will be ecstatic and you will thank yourself for having made the effort to lose the weight that you always dread.

It will obviously be tough in the beginning and you will wonder if your efforts will pay off at all. But these doubts are only natural and you must learn to conquer your fears.

Expect to go through all kinds of questions in your mind. I had all these questions about fasting and no one to answer them. Not a lot of people know the benefits and it's a bit hard to ask people who are uninformed. However, everything I read about fasting proved to be positive. You won't take my word for it because you haven't yet experienced the buzz but read this. It was written by a medical professional and that must be something to take seriously.

"Mattson has also researched the protective benefits of fasting to neurons. If you don't eat for 10–16 hours, your body will go to its fat stores for energy, and fatty acids called ketones will be released into the bloodstream. This has been shown to protect memory and learning functionality, says Mattson, as well as slow disease processes in the brain."

I would say that this is pretty accurate stuff and that my mind is sharper than it used to be. My memory is also better than it used to be. I put it down initially to cutting out junk food but it's more than that. You will begin to feel like a huge cloud has lifted and that you are able to function so much better than you were able to before you started. The results are actually that great! You will not know it unless you experience it firsthand. After all, it is easy to tell others what you went through but it will only give you a clear picture when you experience it yourself. I even went into meditation as something to distract me from thinking about food and that led to a whole new area of development especially since my mind was a lot clearer than it used to be.

Will you go through regrets?

That all depends upon the attitude with which you approach your fasting regime. I went into it with my eyes open. I chose hours when I didn't eat much anyway and it didn't seem to be much of a sacrifice on my part. As my energy levels increased, I found that doing exercise became less of a chore. I made it into fun. For example, how cool is it to stand on the back porch and skip? A jump rope became something that I used quite often and I didn't really cheat on the exercise like some people that I know to have tried fasting. My results were more impressive than theirs so I can only assume that the exercise made the difference. Like that, you have to find things that will help you in small ways but have a big impact on your overall body. You will not realize the benefit unless you pay attention to the many small things that you actually do on a daily basis.

You won't go through regrets if you plan things right and have the right mindset. Since I told myself I wasn't really depriving myself of anything, I didn't find it much different from my everyday life except for those hours between 8 and bedtime. By going to bed earlier, by having an exercise routine and by finding programs on the TV that I enjoyed, I didn't have to think about tucking away the biscuits. It came as second nature to me after a while. I did struggle with motivation for exercising but that was probably because the weather was particularly hot, but in a situation like this, you need to adapt. Walking in the evening was very pleasant, so I changed the time at which I exercised.

So, it is important that you choose something that will fit in well with your schedule and won't allow you to regret it much. If you end up making a schedule and not following through with it then that regret will hound you. So don't make promises that you cannot keep. That regret will learn to outlive any other.

You may have favorite foods that you will miss. It doesn't hurt to have them occasionally and make them really special as long as you don't break your fast. That's the bit where some people find regret. They don't actually want to spend 16 hours without food or cups of milky sugared coffee. Even though you are allowed diet soda, soda is really bad for you and it's probably better to forget all about soda. The amount of sodium that we take into our bodies these days is excessive. But the fact remains that once you give into eating your favorite food, you will feel like eating it over and over again. So your win will lie in not eating it even once.

You may regret choosing the wrong regime to suit your lifestyle. For example, if you regularly eat out with friends in the evening then you may have to adjust the regime to suit your lifestyle. For me, it was easy. I never eat heavily in the evening anyway and wondered why I was so fat. In fact, when I did eat, I tended to choose all the wrong foods and ignore totally my body's need for water. If you are really honest with yourself about your motives and can keep the impetus going, you won't look back and you won't regret what you are doing, because you will be too busy living your life productively to have time for regrets.

Intermittent fasting myths debunked

With any topic, there will be a lot of mysteries and misconceptions. The intermittent fast also has its fair share of myths and in this chapter; we will debunk all of them one by one.

It affects my metabolism

This is the number 1 concern that most people have when it comes to taking **up the** intermittent fast. But it is a misconception, as the fast does not wish to tamper with your metabolic rate at all. It is understood that those with a high metabolic rate will not find it difficult to lose weight and will remain thin. But the job of metabolism is misunderstood and people don't understand what it means to have a good metabolic rate. The main job of this fast is to cut out on the calories and help your body remain fit and healthy for long. So don't worry too much about the metabolism and concentrate on the actual job of the diet.

It will kill muscles

This is the second misconception that most people have when it coms to the intermittent fast. They assume that the diet will cause muscles to weaken, and workouts will further worsen the case. But that is not right. The diet helps in building strong muscles, which will not easily burn. The best routine to take up is the intensity training that will help you avail a strong body and not tire you out easily. However, don't do too much and try to burn excess calories. Keep it limited yet effective.

Eat 5 to 6 meals to remain thin

This misconception has been doing the rounds for quite some time now. There is the theory that eating 5 to 6 meals will help a person lose weight easily. But how can that be possible when the person is constantly filling his body up with food? He or she will not allow the body to burn the calories from the food that he has already eaten. So don't fall into the spiral of eating too many meals a day and stock with the 2 meals a day rule. You will avail its true benefits if you follow a strict schedule.

The diet will affect my sugar

Many people think that this diet is not suitable for those having diabetes or high sugar levels. But the truth remains that the fast will not only help you control your sugar but there have been cases of people having beating illnesses such as diabetes. For that, you have to put in appropriate efforts and ensure that you do all the right things when it comes to the intermittent fast. But it is best to seek medical advice before you take up the fast and do things that will not affect your sugar levels negatively.

It will ignite the starvation mode

Many people don't know what the starvation mode refers to. They wrongly assume that this fast will ignite the starvation mode and their bodies will suffer. The starvation mode comes about when the person starves without food for a long time. Starvation is a state where the body goes into hyper drive and starts storing fat. But this diet will not allow you to starve for more than 20 hours and you will give your body wholesome food after which. So the question of starvation mode being ignited does not come about when the person takes up the intermittent fast.

My diet should be full of proteins

The main goal of the fast is to help the person lose weight and not necessarily build muscles. That is an added need and so, it will come about only if the person puts in the effort to develop lean muscles. As is, the diet incorporates ideal amounts of proteins but if you wish to increase muscle mass then you can increase your protein intake. Eat wholesome foods rich in protein such as white meat and chickpeas and also consume lentils and other such foods rich in proteins.

Breakfast is the most important meal of the day

As you know, breakfast is regarded as the most important meal of the day and your body will suffer if you don't consume breakfast. But this is only a misconception. The breakfast is an optional meal that you can skip when you are following the intermittent fast. It will not impact your body negatively and you can actually lose a lot of weight by planning out your lunch and dinner.

This diet will stress me out

Many people think that the diet will increase the level of cortisol in their body. Here, it is important to understand that cortisol is a good hormone meant to help you beat stress. It is not a bad hormone and you must not think it will harm you. However, the diet will not affect your cortisol levels unless you start worrying about things. If you develop regrets and tensions then the cortisol level will increase and that is independent of the diet. So don't worry about your cortisol increasing and follow the diet in the prescribed manner to derive its full benefits.

Will tire easily on the diet

Tiring out on the diet will occur only if you are over doing it and pushing the limits of your body. If you are fasting for more than 24 hours and working out too much then you will obviously tire out. The key is to strike a fine balance and not overdo it. Remain within your limits and don't over indulge in it.

Heavy lunch and light dinner

This is another misconception that has existed for a long time. Research has shown that the body will burn those carbs better that has been introduced at night. So you will end up burning more fat if you consume the carbs at night as opposed to afternoon. But that doesn't mean you over eat at night.

Everything should be done in limits and you will notice a positive change in no time at all!

Staying put

Now it is obvious that you will feel like abandoning a new diet while starting out owing to its physical demands. But that is only a natural thing, as the human body does not always accept new things easily. For this, you must put in efforts to convince your mind and body that you must stick with it until you see positive changes. In this chapter, we look at the different things that you can do to remain put with your intermittent diet.

Record

The very first thing to do before starting on the diet is recording all your vital statistics. Measure your waist, your arms, thighs, chest and also your weight. Write it down and maintain a thorough record. Now start with the diet and wait for a month before recording again. After that, you must record every fortnight or weekly once. Start comparing it with your previous statistics and you will realize just how much the intermittent fast has worked and how your body is shaping up as per your expectations. Don't stop recording and keep it going for as long as you are practicing the fast.

Reward

Remember to reward yourself from time to time as that is a good way to remain motivated. This reward is not some meal and instead something material such as a fancy camera or a piece of jewelry. You must reward yourself after attaining a milestone. That will ensure that you remain dedicated and motivated. You can also reward yourself a day at the spa or take a vacation. As long as the reward makes you happy, you can take it up. But don't do it too often as it might lose its value over time.

Company

It is always a good idea to ask someone to join in with you when you undertake this fast. It will ensure that the two of you motivate each other and can combined undertake the different rituals that the diet calls for. The ultimate goal is to remain motivated and continue with the diet without giving up on it. But make sure you are not forcing the other person to take it up and they are willfully joining in. the partner can be just about anyone including your spouse, sibling or friend.

Mirror

You can have large full body mirrors installed in your room, which will act as a motivation to you. Human beings love looking at themselves and it is best to visually motivate yourself from time to time. But don't keep looking every second like it is a compulsion. Observe yourself after your work out and you will notice how your body is shaping up, you will feel motivated to keep going and this will help you practice the fast and exercise regularly.

Group

You can look up an intermittent fasting group in your area. Look it up online and join the group. There, you can come face to face with people who have been practicing the fast for some time. They will give you tips on how to maintain the fast and keep going for a long time. You will also remain motivated by joining such a group. If there is no such group in your area then consider starting one yourself. You can get people to join your group and avail benefits. You can hold monthly meetings to instruct them and get them to contribute their experiences while on the diet. This will go a long way in helping you form a large group of dedicated individuals all sharing a common goal.

Visual reminders

Remember to always have visual reminders around you that will tell you to remain motivated and stick with your diet. You can write it down in bold letters and paste it on the wall and other places to remind you about it every now and then. If you are not supposed to eat anything before 1 or 8, then mention that in your phone or make it your computer screen saver. These visual reminders will ensure that you not indulge in your old habits and stick with the diet for good.

Change up the kitchen

The next step is for you to change up your kitchen. Place only fast-related foods and don't fill it up with those that will nullify your fast. Start by clearing everything out. Give it away to soup kitchens and start afresh. Hit the super market to buy only those things that are good for your body. Bring them home and stack them neatly on the kitchen shelves. Your kitchen should look appealing if you wish to remain motivated. If you scatter things around then you will not have the mood to cook and end up ordering take away.

Enjoy food

It is important that you savor the food you consume. Don't think of it as a burden to take up the intermittent fast, as your body will benefit greatly from it. Enjoy whatever food you eat and make sure you don't hate what you eat. Don't deny yourself the occasional cheat meal. You will snap and start binging on it someday, which is a bad thing. Don't do anything in excess and go slow with it. Savor every bite you have and your body will be happy about it and look forward to the next meal.

Carry meals

Remember to carry your own meals to the office or when you step out. Even if you are going to a restaurant, choose to carry your meals with you. You must either cook the meals yourself or have someone prepare a fast meal for you. Introduce variety into it as the same thing every day can get extremely boring and cause you to give up on your fast all too easily. Make it fun for yourself and stick with the fast for a long time.

Remember that you will have to turn the diet into a lifestyle choice so remain put and motivated to continue with it.

Brian Adams

Exercises to build lean muscles

When it comes to building lean muscles, there are certain exercises that you must take up, and train your body to develop strong muscles. These exercises are simple and will not require any heavy equipment. But if you really want to develop strong and lean muscles like a body builder, then you must train at the gym and lift heavy weights.

When you take up these exercises, ensure that you are getting into the right positions, and breathing correctly, as that will contribute towards enhancing your workout regime.

These exercises are all meant to help you tone your body and will aim at specific muscles that you can shape.

Let us start.

Upper body

When it comes to the upper body, you must develop strong muscles in your shoulders, upper arms, chest and abs. These areas are fairly easy to train and let us look at exercise meant for them in particular.

Crunches

When it comes to your abs, you must perform crunches. As you know, crunches are extremely effective and very popular owing to their effectiveness in toning up your stomach muscles. There are many types of crunches but you can perform two that are effective for your upper and lower abs ad also your obliques.

The first one is known as *basic crunch*. The basic crunch is one where you lie on your back and fold your legs such that your knees point to the roof. Now hold your hands across your chest and cross them. Keeping your feet firm on the floor lift up your upper torso and try to touch your knees with your elbows. Many people place their arms behind their head but it is not advisable for you as that can cause injury. Do 10 repetitions and 2 sets. You can increase it after a while.

The second crunch is known as the *bicycle crunch*. As the name suggests, this type requires you to perform crunches like you are riding a bicycle. Lie flat on your back and bring your knees to your chest. Place your arms behind your head and interlock the fingers. Now as you lift your upper torso, push back your legs a little. Now turn to your right while bringing your right knee towards your chest and try to touch it with your left elbow. Repeat on the other side. Keep it going and ensure that you get the position right. Breathe in and out consistently. Repeat 10 times and do 2 sets. You can increase the number as you go.

Weighted push ups

Weighted push-ups will target your shoulders, arms and lower back. It is best to perform this after your crunches. To perform a weighted push up, start by lying on the floor with your face down. Now use your arms to push yourself up in the upper plank position. While there, ask your accomplice to place a weight on your back. This weight needs to be stable and should not move around as that can cause injury. Now start performing a push up and ensure that the weight is placed equally over your entire back.

Plate pinches

The next area to target is your biceps and triceps. As you know, these are muscles present in your upper arms. When you work on these, your arms will start to look well developed. Plate pinches is a fairly easy exercise to perform. You don't have to put in a lot of effort for it. Start by choosing two plates of your choice. They both need to be of the same thickness and weight. Now pinch them together and lift them up and then lower them down. Lift again and lower again. Now pass it to the other hand and do the same. Do as many as feel comfortable.

Chin ups

As you know, it is not enough for you to do just one bicep exercise and it is important that you do at least 2 per muscle. Chin-ups are great for your biceps and will tone them up instantly. Start by choosing a high rod and grab it tightly with both your hands. Your grip should be firm. Have sufficient gap between your palms. Now lift yourself up and try to touch the rod with your chin. Do as many as is comfortable for you.

Lower body exercises

Just like your upper body, your lower body too needs to develop strong muscles. For that, you must take up area specific exercises that will help you tone the muscles present in your lower body.

Lunge walk

Lunge walk is a lower body exercise that will help you maintain strong hip and thigh muscles. It is a rejuvenating type of walk and will help you have strong legs. Start by standing in one place. Place your hands over your hips. Now bend a little and place your right leg in front to get into the lunge position. Next, join your feet together. Now place your left leg in front and bend a little again.

Keep walking that way and ensure that your body feels relaxed. It is best to choose a large field to perform this exercise and keep walking in a straight line. To add to this exercise, you can hold weights in your hand and push your hand up and down every time you get in and out of the lunge position.

Leg raises

Leg raises are meant to help you attain fitter thighs. Start by sleeping on the floor. Now turn to the side and support your upper torso with your forearms. Now lift your right leg mid air and hold it there for some time. To make it tougher, you must lift your left leg as well. Remember that your right leg should not go all the way down and should be lifted and lowered in mid air.

Back leg raises

Back leg raises refer to raising legs to firm up the calves. Start by standing straight and then place your hands on the table or bench. Bend forward and raise your right leg. Point towards the roof and lower again. Repeat it with your other leg. Keep doing this until your legs firm up.

Twist jump

Twist jump is good for your legs and waist. Start by standing straight and then jump normally. Now twist your hips every time you jump up. You should land down with a different hip turned every time. Keep jumping until you feel like your legs and hips are completely exercised.

Squats

Squats are best for your calves. Stand straight and interlock your fingers. Stretch your hands in front of you. Now spread your legs a little and start squatting. Squat once and then rise up again. Do it for 2 minutes. Now do the 4, 3, 2 and 1 method. Here, you have to count to 4 and then lower yourself with every successive count. You must then raise yourself the same way. Next do the same for a count of 3 then 2 then 1.

Remember to always do 10 minutes of warm up before your workouts. You need to warm up the different muscles in your body otherwise you might end up with an injury.

Apart from these, you must also indulge in sports activities such as swimming, jogging, running and jumping. These will contribute towards toning your body and ensure that your heart health is maintained. If you don't know how to incorporate these into your lifestyle then consider accompanying your children when they go out to play a sport like basketball and play like a professional player.

There is also a routine known as the cross fit training. This technique helps you derive the benefits of interval training and also tones up your body. There are certain workout types like TRAN that you can take up and practice regularly.

Brian Adams

Yoga postures for lean muscles

Apart from your exercise routine, you must also practice some yoga postures to help your body avail an internal massage.

In this chapter, we will look at some yoga postures that will help you build strong and lean muscles.

Bridge pose

The first pose to try is the bridge pose. This pose is great for your abs and lower back and also works your butt muscles. To perform this, start by lying flat on your back. Fold your knees and try to pull the heels as close to your butt as possible with the help of your hands. Now lift up your lower torso and butt into the air and allow it to remain mid air. Breathe out when you do so. Place your hands under your body and interlock your fingers. Now lower yourself back down and lift up again. Continue doing so until you tire out.

Boat pose

The next pose to take up is the boat pose. For this, you must balance your body weight on your butt. Start by sitting with a straight back and your legs stretched out in front of you. Now lift your leg up and as high as you can and bend backwards slightly. Now extend your hands on either side of your legs and pull yourself forward. Maintain this pose for a couple of seconds and then place your legs back down. Lift again and repeat pose. You can do this as many times as feel comfortable.

Tree pose

Tree pose is a unique and effective yoga pose for your entire body. It will help your balance and also massage your leg muscles. To get into this pose, start by standing straight. Now place the bottom of your right foot on the inner side of your left thigh. Maintain a straight back and try to balance yourself. Now lift your hands above your head and join them mid air. Maintain pose for a few seconds and then place your legs down. Now repeat with your other leg. You can do this until you can stand straight and not lose your balance.

Cobra pose

The cobra pose is great for your lower back and ab muscles. It is a very easy pose to perform and yet a very effective one. To perform this pose, start by lying on the floor face down. Now lift up your upper torso with the help of your arms. Now look upwards as you feel a stretch in your spine. You must feel a stretch in your ab muscles and feel a burn as well. Hold pose, breathe out and go back to your basic position. Now repeat again.

Downward facing dog

Downward facing dog is a good pose for your back and hamstrings. It will completely stretch your spine out. To perform this pose, start by lying face down on the floor. Now stretch your back and limbs. Now place your palms firmly on the floor and your toes tightly pressed against the floor. Push up your upper body using your palms and your lower body using your toes. You must pull your hands in as much as you can and your butt should point to the roof. Now slowly lift your right leg up and then lower it. Repeat pose with your other leg. Maintain the pose for a couple of seconds and release.

Bow pose

After you finish the downward dog pose, start the bow pose. In this pose, you lie on the floor face down. Now lift your legs up and your hands stretched in front of you. Push your hands back and grab your ankles using your fingers. Now push your upper torso backwards while pulling in your legs. Look up. Maintain this pose for as long as feels comfortable. But don't push your body for it. Release and go back to neutral pose.

Forward bend

Sit straight with your spine erect. Stretch out legs in front of you. Now bend forward and try to touch your toes using your fingers. If you are quite flexible then place your head on your knees. This is an easy looking pose but very tough to perform. You will have to loosen your hamstring if you wish to avail the full bend. That will take some time and you must remain persistent. This pose can also be performed while standing where you bend down and try to touch your toes without bending your knees.

Breathing exercise

Breathing exercises are an important part of yoga. There are two main types i.e. Kapalbhati and pranayama. For the first type, sit with your legs folded and a straight back. Place the backs of your palms on your knees and start exhaling rapidly. But don't go too fast, your exhaled breath should be slightly more audible than your inhaled breath. Every time you exhale, hold the breath for a couple of seconds. Pranayama refers to a slow breathing technique that rejuvenates the mind, body and soul. The technique calls for you to sit with a straight back and folded legs. Now close your eyes and take a few deep breaths. Close your right nostril using your thumb and breathe in deeply through your left nostril. Now hold your breath. Next, hold your left nostril tightly and free your right to breathe out. Hold for a few seconds. Breathe in through your right again and close the nostril and exhale through your left. Do this for no more than 15 minutes.

Child pose

The child pose is one where you relax your body and absorb the effects of the rest of the poses. Start by sitting with your legs folded under your butt. Bend forward and stretch your hands out in front of you. Remain in the pose and contract your stomach inwards.

These form the various yoga exercises that you can try out and supplement your fast.

Brian Adams

Foods That Are Best For Weight Loss and Muscle Building

When it comes to taking up the intermittent fast, you have to supplement your regular meals with special ones that incorporate foods meant to help you lose weight. These foods are basic natural ingredients that can be easily incorporated in your diet without you having to change it up completely. Let us look at these fat-blasting ingredients that you can choose from.

Green tea

Green tea is the number 1 fat blasting drink that millions of people worldwide savor. Green tea is nature's gift to mankind and you can lose a lot of weight by consuming it on a regular basis. But make sure you look for the best quality green tea and buy the ones where the leaves are whole and not powdered too much. The powdered variety is extremely mild and you will have to drink a lot more of it if you want to avail its full benefits. Apart from your regular tea, it is also best for you to consume green tea supplements, which will increase your immunity as well. They are available over the counter or you can also buy them online. However, don't over do it and consume many tablets at once to lose weight faster as that will not happen!

Ginger

Ginger is a spice plant extensively grown in Asian countries. It is used in their cuisine and also added to sweets. Ginger is a digestive and aids in breaking down the complex food molecules. So by consuming it, you are making it easier for your liver to break down the food compounds and eliminate the toxins at a faster pace. You can cut it into small pieces and add it to your soups and curries. You can also add it to tea and brew a health potion for yourself. Ginger is easily available at any grocery store and you can easily grow it yourself.

Turmeric

Turmeric is like ginger and grows under soil. It is the tuber that grows next to the root of the plant. Turmeric is a yellow tuber that contains a chemical known as curcumin. This chemical is very beneficial to the human body and can fight cancer, strengthen your bones and increase your immunity. But the main function of curcumin is to help in digestion and aid in weight loss. It literally cuts through the fat in your body and ensures that you remain fit and in perfect health. Just add a little to your curry and you will avail full benefits of this spice.

Flax seeds

When you are trying to lose weight and cut fat from your body, it is very important for you to incorporate as much fiber as possible. This fiber can be availed from your foods and you must choose those that are rich in it. Flax seeds are extremely rich in fiber and will help you eliminate toxins from your body. You have to grind them into a fine powder and add it into water. Now consume this water at night before retiring to bed. Your stomach will be thoroughly cleansed the next morning and you will start feeling lighter. Flax seeds can be easily bought from any departmental store.

Nuts

Just like seeds, nuts are also extremely rich in fiber. You can crush them a bit and add it to warm milk and consume it at night. Just make sure you are not picking those nuts that have a lot of fat in them. You can also munch on a few almonds after every meal, as they will provide your body with all the fiber that you need.

Bottle gourd

Bottle gourd is also an important ingredient that should supplement your weight loss. You can juice it or grate it and add to your salad. It contains a chemical that helps in cutting out the fat in your body. Bottle gourd skin is also good for you so don't peel it before consuming and allow the skin to remain. You can grate it and add a little honey and consume it in the morning. You can grow your own gourd if you like. Again don't over do it in a bid to lose your weight at a rapid pace, which will never work for you!

Pepper

Peppercorn or cayenne pepper are both great for your body. They contain capsaicin, which helps in cutting the fat from your body. It is easy to incorporate this ingredient in your diet. It can be used as a seasoning to sprinkle over your soups and curries. You can also add cayenne pepper to your health tonic and avail its full benefits. Capsaicin is also important for your digestion and will break down the molecules in your foods to make it easier for your liver and gut to digest the food. If you think capsaicin is too hot for you then you can add in a little honey to it.

Ginseng

Ginseng is a naturally occurring substance that is quite beneficial for the human body. It has been used for hundreds of years in China. Ginseng is a root that is dried and consumed to remain healthy. It has active ingredients that prevent the formation of fat in the body. You can add a little ginseng powder to your curries and can also buy supplements from specialty stores or from online stores. But there is a limit to how much you can consume and must remain within your limits.

Noni

Noni is a fruit that is grown in Asia. This fruit is known to fight cancer cells and increase immunity. It will also help you remain slim and fit for long. You can avail it in syrup form and consume it on a daily basis. Make sure you buy genuine syrup and not some untested and spurious tonic. Look for recommendations and then buy it from an online store.

Cumin seeds

Cumin seeds are great for your digestion. They are spices used in Asian cuisine. You can toast them a little to release their flavor and then add them to a coffee grinder to grind into a fine powder. This powder you can sprinkle over your salads and soups. Cumin will effectively cut down on your fat cells and break down food molecules. It is also great to combat flatulence and you can have a clean digestive system by consuming cumin seeds on a regular basis.

Stinging nettle

Stinging nettle is the next natural ingredient to use for your weight loss. The leaves of this plant will sting quite a lot because of their shape. So you must be careful while handling them and ensure that you don't consume it whole. It is best to buy the syrup and consume it. You will reel in its real benefits only if you consume it on a regular basis. The stinging nettle is should be consumed sparingly and don't over dose on it to try and lose weight fast.

Cardamom

Cardamom seeds are great for digestion. You must pound it into a fine powder and add it to your soups and salads. You can also consume the seeds whole with a little water. It will also aid in weight loss and help you maintain an ideal weight. It is slightly sweet in flavor and will leave behind a fresh taste in your mouth. So consider chewing on some seeds after your meal.

Although most of these are safe to consume without medical advice, it is best to consult your doctor before consuming any of the supplements. This is especially important if you are a pregnant or nursing woman or a senior citizen. You must also observe due precaution while administering it to children.

Brian Adams

What Not To Do While On The Fast

When you take up the intermittent fast, you must do certain things that will supplement it and along with those, you must avoid doing certain things, as they can be bad for your fast.

In this chapter, we will look at the various things that you must avoid doing in order to help you with your diet.

Smoking

Smoking is a bad habit that you must avoid when on the diet. It might end up countering the good effects of your diet and retard your progress. I know it will be difficult for you to stop smoking all of a sudden and so, it is best that you take it slow. Consider availing help to kick the habit and join a rehab program. You can also have visual reminders placed around you that ask you to not smoke.

Drinking

Just like smoking, you must also not drink. Drinking alcohol can hamper your progress. Alcohol has molecules that are difficult for your liver to break down and it will get confused. You will end up countering the good that your diet is doing to your body. It's fine to have an occasional drink at the dinner table but don't go all out and empty an entire bottle. The choice of drink also matters so choose something that is not sugary and is good for your body when consumed in small quantities. Ask your friends and family members to not force you and tell them clearly that you have stopped drinking.

Junk foods

Junk foods are your fast's worst enemies. I know that it is common to think that you are now eating healthy foods and sticking to a set timetable, so it is fine for you to indulge in some junk food binging. But that is an absolutely wrong idea to develop and follow and your junk food binge will only cause you to go back on your fast. Most other experts will ask you to have your favorite fast food once in a while but it is best that you completely avoid it. It is a good idea to prepare healthy alternatives at home. Look up recipes of your favorite junk foods and substitute all the bad ingredients with nutritious ones. For example, you can make a wheat-based pizza crust and top it with fresh vegetables.

Sedentary lifestyle

Remember that having a sedentary lifestyle is not acceptable when you take up the intermittent fast diet. You have to remain as active as possible and indulge in one physical activity or the other. We looked at the different sports activities that you can take up for yourself and why they will prove to be good to build strong and lean muscles. You must consider exercise part of your diet and use it to sculpt your body into a desirable shape and make use of the yoga postures to keep your internal organs well oiled and massaged.

Over reading

Don't go on a mission to uncover the 100 secrets of the diet. People tend to over read about something and feel disappointed when they come across some unpleasant articles. You surely don't need to know about them and it is best that you limit your research. It is fine to read on the different things that the diet can do for you but going in the wrong direction is not advisable. Read in limit and only from reliable sites and sources.

Assuming

When it comes to certain aspects of the diet like the 16-hour gap and skipping meals understand why it is beneficial and don't simply do whatever you like. Don't assume that any type of fast will work for you and end up starving yourself. Intermittent fasting does not mean starving so ensure that you do all the right things for the fast to work well for you.

Taking long break

When you start on a diet, it will be a good idea to complete a course and then decide to take a break from it. This break is important, as your body will have to distinguish your fasting phase from your non-fasting phase. But don't take too long a break and limit it to no more than a week's time. If you think a break is unnecessary then don't take it at all. It is not obligatory but taking a short break will allow you to see how beneficial the fast really is.

Media influence

Don't get influenced by what you see around you or read. There will be several fake stories planted to get you hooked on to the fast and also promise you a lean and slim body within a short period of time. But you have to be wise and understand that the fast will take a little time to show results. Don't get fooled by such gimmicks and stay away from those that try to sell you products by claiming it will help with your diet. The only thing that can help you with your diet is your dedication alone and nothing else.

Giving up

Giving up on the fast is never an option for you. It might take some time for it to show results but you must not lose hope. Regardless of how fat and unfit you are, the fast will definitely help you and give away positive results. It's a matter of a few weeks and remaining patient all through out. Just make sure that you are following the correct steps.

Brian Adams

Key takeaway

The very first thing to do is understand what the intermittent fast stands for. If you confuse it with dieting then you will end up making mistakes. Take I slow and understand everything that there is to about the diet. As you know, the diet is not a diet and just a diet schedule for you to follow. Do your own research and don't rely on what you hear from others. Put in efforts to read about the diet from reliable sources and avoid getting information from dubious sources.

This book attempted to give you an in depth analysis of the diet and tell you about the different aspects of the diet. You can read the book over and over again and understand everything carefully. Focus on the main chapters like why the fast works and how you can come up with a plan to follow the diet on a daily basis.

The main idea of the diet is to cut out on the amount of calories that you consume in a day. Start by cutting it by 3/4ths and then ½ and then quarter, but this is only possible if you calculate how many calories you intake and then reduce it slowly. You must also cut out on 2 meals a day preferably the breakfast and snack.

As you know, there are many forms of intermittent diets and you must choose the best one for yourself. That decision is for you to make and you must choose the one that will help you attain your diet goals fastest. You can take the help of a dietician if required and ask them to suggest to you the best form of diet to take up.

You must adhere to the intermittent fasting protocols when you wish to take it up. Make sure you are doing things that are as per the basic rules of the diet. Regardless of whether you choose the 16-hour, 20 hour or 24-hour routine, you must follow the rules and understand the various pros and cons of each before taking it up.

There are certain things that you must do to supplement your diet that include eating all the best ingredients that you can get your hands on. For this, you must buy fresh fruits and vegetables and other condiments that are certified by the diet. I have provided a list in this book and you must choose your ingredients from it. Visit the super market twice a month and get everything in bulk.

Get rid of all the unhealthy foods in your house and arrange the good foods in a neat manner to help you remain motivated.

The next thing to incorporate is exercise routines that will help you burn away the excess calories present in the body. It is this routine that will help you remain fit and active when you take up the diet. The various exercise routines that you can take up have been explained in this book and you can use it as a blue print to formulate your exercise routine. But don't over exercise and try to calculate how many calories you must burn in a day.

The diet helps the human body in many ways. Right from combating illnesses such as cancer and improving heart health, it aids in many ways. It also helps in increasing immunity. If you follow the diet correctly, you can also maintain glowing skin and shiny hair. The diet will also leave you with string teeth and prevent unnecessary conditions. The autophagy will also improve where your cells turn strong and free of damage. You will also have better growth hormone secretion and remain fit and healthy for long.

It will be a little difficult in the beginning but you must try to remain as motivated as possible. Start by having visual reminders to motivate you and then start maintaining a record of your progress. You must also reward yourself for sticking with the fast and ensure that you leave behind all the regrets. Start the fast on a happy note and maintain it for as long as you are on the diet. Don't entertain negative thoughts and remain positive all through your intermittent fasting journey.

You must avoid doing certain things like smoking and drinking, which can reverse the effects of your diet. So try your best to stay as away from these as possible. If you think it is difficult for you to do so then join a rehab or correction center that will help you kick the habit as soon as possible. Yu must also inform your friends and family members about your fast so that they don't force you to eat something that you wish to stay away from, especially having a drink.

Sleeping well is extremely important. When you sleep, your body fixes your internal processes and repairs your body from the inside out. If you don't sleep well then you will end up having a tired body and mind, which will not respond to the diet properly. Try to get 8 straight hours of sleep a night and don't bail on it. If you are finding it difficult to sleep properly then there are many things that you can do like making use of music and scented candles to sleep properly.

There are many precautions that you must observe when you take up the intermittent fast. If you are suffering from an illness then you must ask your doctor if you can start with the diet. If you consume any medicines regularly then you must stick with a routine and not allow the diet to affect it. The diet should also be modified for young children and senior citizens.

Brian Adams

Conclusion

I thank you once again for choosing this book and hope you had a good time reading it. The main aim of this book was to educate you on the process of intermittent fasting. As you know now, the fast is not a diet and is just a diet schedule for you to improve your body's functioning.

Intermittent fasting can have some extremely positive benefits for those who are trying to drop some body fat and lose weight as well as build up muscles and strength. Men and women will react differently to the intermittent fasting because their bodies work differently and each individual will show different results. Experimentation is the key here; experiment to find out what works and what doesn't for you.

There are loads of ways to do intermittent fasting, including:

- A regular fast and feast. Fast for a set number of hours and then eat all of your daily calories in a set time span. Most people prefer to do a 16-hour fasting as it has been scientifically established that it will work for anyone and every one. However, if there is another type of diet that you think will suit you then you can take that up as well without hesitating too much.

- Eat as normal but fast 1 or 2 times a week. Eat your normal meals every day but pick a couple of days when you can easily fast for a 24-hour period. Perhaps, eat your evening meal on a Sunday and then don't eat again until the following evening.

Just fast occasionally. This is the best way for those who don't want to work too hard at this but want to lose a bit of their body fat. Just skip out a meal whenever it suits you. Perhaps you don't really have time for breakfast, skip it. If you pig out on Saturday, don't eat anything again until Sunday evening.

Figure out what works for you

You have absolutely nothing to lose by giving this a try. It will not hurt your health to skip a meal or two or to go 24 hours without eating. Try it; you might actually find that it's a way of life you can live with. Do research it first before you dismiss it out of hand. It does work but it won't work for everyone.

After all, you have to love your body enough to know that change needs to be brought in. Imagine what would happen to it if you stop caring about your body. You will have to live with the guilt of not taking the opportunity and helping your body recuperate and establish a strong metabolic rate. It is always better to start early so that, you have the time to adjust to the diet. Your body might not be able to take too much at once and you have to take it slow if you wish to make this a lasting habit.

I must add this – if you have diabetes, hypoglycemia or any other disease or condition that affects your blood sugar, you must seek medical advice before you start an intermittent fasting program.

I hope that I have been able to shed some light on intermittent fasting for you. This is just the basics of it and I urge you to do more research on whichever method you choose to make sure it is right for you and, if necessary, speak to your doctor first.

And remember, above all, this is not a diet; it is a way of life

Brian Adams

Achieve Your Next Level Health:

Low Carb: Ketogenic Diet to Overcome Belly Fat, Lose Pounds, and Live Healthy

Health and Fitness: Uncommon HIGH Impact Quick Wins You Should Start Today - Nutrition, Natural Health, and Healthy Living

Detox: Cleanse for Fast Weight Loss, Anti Aging, Holistic Healing and Better Health

Vegan: Vegan Diet for Easy Weight Loss and Healthy Living Through Natural Foods

Other Recommended Books to Become More Effective and Fulfilled In Life:

Self Improvement: Self Discipline - An Uncommon Guide to Instant Self Control, Incredible Willpower, and Insane Productivity

Spirit Guides: Ultimate Guide to Exploring the Spirit World, Finding Your Angel Guide and Mastering Spirit Communication

Brian Adams

www.ingramcontent.com/pod-product-compliance
Lightning Source LLC
Chambersburg PA
CBHW071043290526
45795CB00004B/1292